NURSING ANATOMY AND PHYSIOLOGY Q & A

BY

ALFAJIRI PUBLISHERS

ALFAJIRI PUBLICATIONS
1510 WEST PAWNEE
WICHITA, KANSAS

Table of contents

Cardiovascular system

Digestive System

MUSCULAR SYSTEM

SKELETAL SYSTEM

Endocrine System

Circulatory system

FINAL

Medical Root words

Cardiovascular system

QUIZ 1

1. Blood returning to the heart from the inferior vena cava would enter the:

a. left atrium
b. right atrium
c. left ventricle
d. right ventricle

2. Blood in the pulmonary arteries:

a. enters the heart's right ventricle
b. is heading towards the lungs
c. leaves the left ventricle to enter the aorta
d. flows from the lungs towards the heart's left atrium

3. Fetal blood would bypass the pulmonary circuit by flowing through this structure located in the fetal interatrial wall:

a. the tricuspid atrioventricular valve
b. the ductus arteriosus
c. the foramen ovale
d. the pulmonary semilunar valve
e. the aortic semilunar valve

4. Located between the right atrium and right ventricle is the:

a. tricuspid atrioventricular valve
b. bicuspid/mitral atrioventricular valve
c. fossa ovalis
d. pulmonary semilunar valve
e. aortic semilunar valve

5. The pulmonary veins:

a. carry oxygenated blood away from the heart
b. carry oxygenated blood towards the heart

c. carry deoxygenated blood away from the heart
d. carry deoxygenated blood towards the heart

6. Which of the following statements about veins is CORRECT?

a. venous valves are an extension of the tunica media
b. up to one third of the total blood volume is stored in the venous circulation at any given time
c. veins have a small lumen in relation to the thickness of its wall
d. the flow of venous blood is not a major result of one's blood pressure

7. Peripheral resistance of blood vessels:

a. decreases as the length of the blood vessel increases
b. increases as the diameter of the blood vessel increases
c. increases as the viscosity of blood increases
d. does not play a major role in affecting one's blood pressure

8. Blood flow to the skin:

a. is regulated mainly by a decreasing pH
b. increases when external environmental temperature rises
c. increases when internal body temperature decreases so that the skin does not freeze
d. is not an important source of nutrients and oxygen for skin cells

9. Which of the following statements about the movement of materials at the 'systemic' capillary level is CORRECT?

a. oxygen is actively transported up its concentration gradient
b. waste products such as CO_2 follow the same general pathway as O_2
c. CO_2 moves from its site of production into the interstitial fluid
d. if capillary blood osmotic pressure is much greater than interstitial fluid osmotic pressure, tissue edema will likely result

10. Which arterial tunic modification is most responsible for maintaining blood pressure?

a. a thin tunica interna/intima
b. a thick tunica media
c. a thin tunica externa
d. a thick tunica adventitia

ANSWERS

	4. A	8. B
1. B	5. B	9. C
2. B	6. D	10. B
3. C	7. C	

QUIZ 2

1. Normally, blood leaving the right ventricle immediately flows through the:

a. tricuspid atrioventricular valve

b. bicuspid/mitral atrioventricular valve

c. ileocecal valve

d. pulmonary semilunar valve

e. aortic semilunar valve

2. Blood leaving the left atrium normally immediately flows through the:

a. tricuspid atrioventricular valve

b. bicuspid/mitral atrioventricular valve

c. ileocecal valve

d. pulmonary semilunar valve

e. aortic semilunar valve

3. Deoxygenated blood is normally found only:

a. in the heart's atria

b. in the heart's ventricles

c. in the right side of the heart

d. in the left side of the heart

4. Closing of the _____ normally prevents backflow of blood into the left ventricle:

a. tricuspid atrioventricular valve

b. bicuspid/mitral atrioventricular valve

c. ileocecal valve

d. pulmonary semilunar valve

e. aortic semilunar valve

5. Closing of the _____ normally prevents backflow of blood into the right ventricle:

a. tricuspid atrioventricular valve

b. bicuspid/mitral atrioventricular valve

c. ileocecal valve

d. pulmonary semilunar valve

e. aortic semilunar valve

6. The influence of a blood vessel's diameter on peripheral resistance is:

a. minimal since the diameter of a blood vessel's lumen only has a minor effect on peripheral resistance

b. very large since peripheral resistance is directly influenced by the diameter of a blood vessel's lumen

c. very small since the diameter of the lumen of a blood vessel does not vary

d. very large since the greater the diameter of the lumen of a blood vessel, the greater amount of peripheral resistance will be present

7. When evaluating the dynamics of capillary blood flow, capillary blood hydrostatic pressure:

a. does not play a role

b. is generally greater at the arterial end of a capillary than its venous end

c. forces fluid from the interstitial spaces into the capillary

d. is usually equal to and canceled out by capillary blood osmotic pressure

8. Which of the following structures are directly involved in the "pulmonary circuit"?

a. superior vena cava, right atrium and left ventricle

b. right ventricle, pulmonary arteries and left atrium

c. left ventricle, aorta and inferior vena cava

d. right atrium, aorta and left ventricle

9. Which of the following structures are directly involved in the "systemic circuit"?

a. superior vena cava, right ventricle and left ventricle

b. right ventricle, pulmonary arteries and left atrium

c. left ventricle, aorta and inferior vena cava

d. right atrium, pulmonary trunk and left ventricle

10. Histologically, the _____ is simple squamous epithelium surrounded by a sparse connective tissue layer:

a. tunica interna/intima

b. tunica media

c. tunica externa

d. tunica adventitia

ANSWERS

1. D

2. B

3. C

4. E

5. D

6. B

7. B

8. B

9. C

10. A

QUIZ 3

1. The lining of the inner walls of the heart's chambers is termed the:

a. visceral pericardium

b. serous pericardium

c. epicardium

d. myocardium

e. endocardium

2. The outermost layer of the heart's serous pericardium is termed the:

a. visceral pericardium

b. parietal pericardium

c. epicardium

d. myocardium

e. endocardium

3. The heart's natural pacemaker is termed the:

a. sinoatrial node

b. atrioventricular node

c. bundle of His/atrioventricular bundle

d. left and right bundle branches

e. Purkinje fibers

4. The heart's electrical conduction network found within the ventricular myocardium is termed the:

a. sinoatrial node

b. atrioventricular node

c. bundle of His/atrioventricular bundle

d. left and right bundle branches

e. Purkinje fibers

5. If the heart's natural pacemaker fails to fire, then:

a. no blood would enter the atria

b. no blood would enter the ventricles

c. the node on the floor of the right atrium would act as a secondary pacemaker

d. the node on the floor of the left ventricle would act as a secondary pacemaker

e. the person would die within minutes

6. Which tunic of an artery contains endothelium?

a. tunica interna/intima

b. tunica media

c. tunica externa

d. tunica adventitia

7. The exchange of gases and nutrients between blood and tissues is a major function of:

a. arterioles

b. arteries

c. capillaries

d. veins

8. Which of the following statements best describes arteries?

a. all arteries carry oxygenated blood towards the heart

b. all arteries contain valves to prevent the back-flow of blood

c. all arteries carry blood away from the heart

d. only large arteries are lined with endothelium

9. The circulatory pathway that carries blood from the digestive tract towards the liver is termed the:

a. coronary circuit

b. cerebral circuit

c. hepatic portal circuit

d. pulmonary circuit

10. Immediately following strenuous and vigorous exercise, which of the following is most likely to occur?

a. blood will be rapidly diverted to the digestive organs

b. the skin will be cold and clammy

c. capillaries of the active muscles will be engorged with blood

d. blood flow to the kidneys quickly increases

ANSWERS

1. E

2. B

3. A

4. E

5. C

6. A

7. C

8. C

9. C

10. C

QUIZ 4

1. Sympathetic stimulation to the heart's natural pacemaker normally results in:

a. a faster heart rate

b. a greater force of myocardial contraction

c. both choices (a) and (b) are correct

d. the heart's natural pacemaker is not influenced by sympathetic stimulation

2. The normal heart sounds (lub and dup) are produced by which of the following events?

a. sympathetic stimulation of the sinoatrial node

b. closure of the atrioventricular and semilunar valves

c. friction of blood flowing against the chamber walls

d. ventricular systole

3. Following a motor vehicle accident, a large loss of blood will initially cause:

a. a lowered BP due to a decreased cardiac output

b. a higher BP due to an increased stroke volume

c. no change in BP but a slower heart rate

d. no change in BP but an increased respiration rate

4. The left ventricle's myocardium is thicker than the right ventricle's myocardium in order to:

a. accommodate a greater volume of blood

b. increase the size of the thoracic cavity during diastole

c. contract with a greater pressure

d. force blood through a smaller semilunar valve

5. The pain associated with decreased blood delivery to the heart's tissues, possibly caused by a transient spasm of coronary arteries, is termed:

a. ischemia

b. myocardial infarction

c. pericarditis

d. angina pectoris

6. A thrombus in the first branch off the aortic arch would affect the flow of blood to the:

a. left side of the head and neck, and left upper arm

b. myocardium

c. left upper arm

d. right side of the head and neck, and right upper arm

7. At the Battle of Shiloh during the American Civil War, Confederate General Albert Johnston was killed when he was shot in the back of the knee and rapidly bled to death. Which blood vessel was most likely to have been injured?

a. femoral artery

b. common iliac artery

c. anterior tibialis artery

d. popliteal artery

8. Which of the following is NOT generally considered part of the Circle of Willis?

a. anterior cerebral artery

b. posterior cerebral artery

c. anterior communicating artery

d. posterior communicating artery

e. vertebral artery

9. The longest superficial vein in the body is the:

a. right brachial vein

b. left radial vein

c. superior vena cava

d. great saphenous vein

e. anterior tibialis vein

10. An external iliac artery empties into the:

a. common iliac artery

b. internal iliac artery

c. abdominal aorta

d. femoral artery

e. renal artery

ANSWERS

1. A

2. B

3. A

4. C

5. D

6. D

7. D

8. E

9. D

10. D

QUIZ 5

1. Stenosis of the bicuspid/mitral atrioventricular valve may initially cause an increase of pressure in the:

a. superior and inferior venae cavae

b. left ventricle

c. pulmonary circuit

d. coronary circuit

2. If an abnormally increased amount of connective tissue were to form connecting together the serous visceral and parietal pericardium, which of the following events would most likely result?

a. strengthening of the frail pericardial layers with an improvement of cardiac function

b. decreased fluid production in the pericardial cavity since it is no longer necessary

c. interference with the heart's normal mechanical activity

d. decreased friction between the visceral and parietal pericardial layers

3. Which of the following statements about cardiac output is CORRECT?

a. stroke volume can increase when the end diastolic volume decreases

b. if a semilunar valve was partially obstructed, then the end systolic volume in the affected ventricle would decrease

c. a decreased venous return will cause an increased end diastolic volume

d. a decreased heart rate will cause an increased end diastolic volume

4. The coronary vessel external to the heart that empties blood into the right atrium is the:

a. superior vena cava

b. inferior vena cava

c. coronary sinus

d. all of the above choices (a, b and c) are correct

5. The left ventricle is serviced by all of the following coronary vessels, EXCEPT the:

a. left coronary artery

b. anterior interventricular artery, (also known as left anterior descending artery)

c. marginal artery

d. circumflex artery

6. Increased end-systolic volume results in:

a. more blood ejected from the ventricle per beat

b. higher cardiac output

c. more blood remaining in the ventricle after contraction

d. higher end-diastolic volume

7. The superior vena cava drains all of the following organs, EXCEPT the:

a. arms

b. shoulders

c. abdomen

d. head

e. neck

8. An excessively shortened PR-interval can have this effect on cardiac output (CO):

a. decrease CO because it reduces ventricular contraction time

b. decrease CO because it reduces ventricular fill time

c. increase CO because it increases force of ventricular contraction

d. increase CO because it increases end-diastolic volume

9. An abnormal clot within a blood vessel that breaks loose and now travels in the blood is termed:

a. a thrombus

b. an aneurysm

c. an embolus

d. a cerebrovascular accident

10. Increase in afterload in the aorta can have what effect on cardiac output (CO):

a. increase CO because of increased blood pressure and blood volume

b. increase CO because of increased elastic recoil of the aorta

c. decrease CO because of increased backpressure opposing ventricular ejection of blood

d. decrease CO because of increased hydrostatic pressure and increased stroke volume

ANSWERS

1. C
2. C
3. A
4. C
5. C
6. C
7. C
8. B
9. C
10. C

Digestive System

QUIZ 1

1. The main functions of the digestive system are
- A) ingestion and digestion
- B) propulsion and secretion
- C) absorption and elimination
- D) all of the above

2. The movement of digestion products, electrolytes, vitamins, and water across the GI tract epithelium and into the underlying blood and lymphatic vessels is called
- A) ingestion
- B) absorption
- C) digestion
- D) secretion

3. All of the following are organs of the digestive system except the
- A) spleen
- B) liver
- C) tongue
- D) esophagus

4. Which selection includes only accessory digestive organs?
- A) salivary glands, thyroid gland, pancreas, liver
- B) stomach, duodenum, pancreas, gallbladder
- C) gallbladder, liver, pancreas, salivary glands
- D) liver, thyroid gland, gallbladder, spleen

5. Movements in the small intestine that churn the materials being digested and mix them with intestinal secretions are called

A) peristalsis

B) pendular motility

C) segmentation

D) haustral churning

6. Which term describes the wave of muscular contraction that moves material through the GI tract toward the anus?

A) peristalsis

B) pendular motility

C) segmentation

D) haustral churning

7. Digestive functions of the tongue include

A) manipulating and mixing ingested materials during chewing

B) helping compress partially digested food to form a bolus

C) assisting in the swallowing process

D) all of the above

8. The three pairs of multicellular salivary glands that secrete into the oral cavity are the _____ glands.

A) alpha, beta, and gamma

B) parotid, submandibular, and sublingual

C) palatine, lingual, and pharyngeal

D) serous, mucous, and mixed

9. What is the mineralized matrix, similar to bone but harder, that forms the primary mass of each tooth?

A) enamel

B) dentin

C) cementum

D) pulp

10. Which selection does not correctly pair a type of tooth with its description?

A) incisors, one or two roots and spoon-shaped

B) canines, one root and conical with a pointed tip

C) premolars, one or two roots and flat crowns with cusps

D) molars, three or more roots and large, broad, flat crowns

11. Which mesentery covers most of the abdominal organs, extending inferiorly like an apron from the greater curvature of the stomach?

A) mesentery proper

B) lesser omentum

C) greater omentum

D) mesocolon

12. From deep to superficial, what are the tunics of the intraperitoneal portions of the GI tract?

A) serosa, muscularis, submucosa, and mucosa

B) mucosa, submucosa, muscularis, and serosa

C) adventitia, muscularis, submucosa, and mucosa

D) mucosa, submucosa, muscularis, and adventitia

13. In which of the following selections are the GI tract organs or regions correctly matched with the type of epithelium that lines them?

A) oral cavity and esophagus; stratified cuboidal

B) stomach and small intestine; stratified squamous

C) cecum, colon, and rectum; simple columnar

D) all of the above

14. Within the mucous membrane of the GI tract, the layer of areolar connective tissue is called the

A) mucosal lining

B) lamina propria

C) muscularis mucosae

D) submucosa

15. Which tunic of the GI tract typically contains an inner circular layer and an outer longitudinal layer, with the myenteric nerve plexus in between?

    A)   muscularis

    B)   mucosa

    C)   submucosa

    D)   adventitia

16. The esophagus enters the abdominal cavity through an opening in the diaphragm, the _____, before it connects to the stomach.

    A)   diaphragmatic foramen

    B)   thoracic canal

    C)   cardiac orifice

    D)   esophageal hiatus

17. Histological features of the esophageal wall include

    A)   a mucosa lined with stratified cuboidal epithelium

    B)   submucosal glands that produce a thin, watery fluid

    C)   a single layer of skeletal muscle in the muscularis

    D)   an outer fibrous layer, the adventitia, with no serosa

18. What are the three phases of the swallowing process?

    A)   mastication, eruption, and dentition

    B)   oral, cranial, and pharyngeal

    C)   voluntary, pharyngeal, and esophageal

    D)   cardiac, gastric, and pyloric

19. Which digestive organ mechanically and chemically transforms a food bolus into chyme?

    A)   esophagus

    B)   stomach

    C)   small intestine

    D)   large intestine

20. Which list proceeds from the superior to the inferior end of the stomach?

    A)   pylorus, fundus, cardia, body

    B)   cardia, body, fundus, pylorus

    C)   cardia, fundus, body, pylorus

    D)   body, cardia, pylorus, fundus

21. The prominent folds of the mucosa that nearly disappear when the stomach expands are the

    A)   gastric pits

    B)   rugae

    C)   plicae

    D)   omenta

22. From the superior end downward, the three segments of the small intestine are the

    A)   ileum, duodenum, and jejunum

    B)   duodenum, jejunum, and ileum

    C)   jejunum, ileum, and duodenum

    D)   duodenum, ileum, and jejunum

23. What is the function of the villi in the small intestine?

    A)   to decrease the amount of exposed surface

    B)   to facilitate enzyme retention and dispersal

    C)   to increase the surface area for absorption and secretion

    D)   to sweep particles across the surface with wavelike actions

24. Which sequence lists the regions of the large intestine in order, from the end of the ileum to the anus?

    A)   cecum, rectum, anal canal, colon

    B)   colon, rectum, anal canal, cecum

    C)   cecum, colon, rectum, anal canal

    D)   colon, cecum, rectum, anal canal

25. Arrange the segments of the colon in the sequence through which digested material passes prior to defecation: (1) sigmoid (2) transverse (3) descending (4) ascending

   A)   4, 2, 3, 1

   B)   2, 1, 4, 3

   C)   1, 3, 4, 2

   D)   3, 1, 2, 4

26. The mucosa of the large intestine is characterized by

   A)   lack of intestinal villi

   B)   numerous goblet cells and intestinal glands

   C)   many lymphatic nodules and cells in the lamina propria

   D)   all of the above

27. Production of bile is one of several important functions of the

   A)   gallbladder

   B)   liver

   C)   pancreas

   D)   small intestine

28. Bile is stored and concentrated in the

   A)   gallbladder

   B)   liver

   C)   biliary apparatus

   D)   duodenum

29. Which hormones stimulate the production of pancreatic juice and bicarbonate?

   A)   angiotensin and epinephrine

   B)   gastrin and insulin

   C)   cholecystokinin and secretin

   D)   insulin and glucagon

30. Age-related changes in the digestive system include which of the following?

   A)   reduced secretion of mucin, enzymes, and acid

B) decreased replacement of epithelial cells

C) diminished muscular tone and GI tract motility

D) all of the above

ANSWERS

28. A

1. D   29. C

2. B   30. D

3. B

4. C

5. C

6. A

7. D

8. B

9. B

10. A

11. C

12. B

13. C

14. B

15. A

16. D

17. D

18. C

19. B

20. C

21. B

22. B

23. C

24. C

25. A

26. D

27. B

QUIZ 2

1.

On each maxilla and each side of the mandible, both the deciduous and permanent dentitions typically include two _____ for slicing or cutting into food.

    A)   incisors

    B)   canines

    C)   premolars

    D)   molars

2

Unique to the permanent dentition, the two pairs of _____ on each jaw are used for crushing and grinding food.

    A)   canines

    B)   premolars

    C)   molars

    D)   wisdom teeth

3

Which statement does not accurately describe an aspect of swallowing?

    A)   first phase occurs in oral cavity and involves the tongue and hard palate

    B)   actions are primarily involuntary until the bolus reaches the oropharynx

    C)   soft palate, uvula, and pharyngeal constrictors participate in second phase

    D)   third phase involves involuntary control of both skeletal and smooth muscle

4

Which salivary glands empty into the oral cavity through single ducts on each side of the lingual frenulum, posterior to the incisors?

    A)   parotid

    B)   sublingual

    C)   submandibular

D) all of the above

5

Which salivary glands are located subcutaneously, offering a good environment for a once-common childhood virus that is now largely controlled by vaccination?

A) parotid

B) sublingual

C) submandibular

D) all of the above

6

Submucosal nerve plexus is to submucosa as _____ nerve plexus is to muscularis.

A) autonomic

B) myenteric

C) Meissner

D) celiac

7

Histologically, the stomach mucosa comprises

A) a simple columnar epithelial lining, with numerous gastric pits

B) goblet cells that secrete a thick carpet of mucin over the surface

C) an extra, inner layer of smooth muscle called the oblique layer

D) all of the above

8

The _____ is actually composed of _____ peritoneum and is therefore found only on organs within the peritoneal cavity.

A) lesser omentum; visceral

B) mesentery proper; visceral

C) adventitia; parietal

D) serosa; visceral

9

Portions of the GI tract outside the peritoneal cavity are surrounded by a layer of areolar connective tissue called the

- A) adventitia
- B) serosa
- C) mucosa externa
- D) tunica albuginea

10

Which selection correctly pairs a type of gastric epithelial cell with its secretion?

- A) mucous neck cell, alkaline mucin
- B) parietal cell, pepsinogen
- C) enteroendocrine cell, somatostatin
- D) chief cell, hydrochloric acid

11

The production of acid and enzymes by the gastric mucosa can be controlled by

- A) sympathetic innervation
- B) parasympathetic innervation
- C) hormones from the mucosa itself
- D) all of the above

12

Which hormone, produced by enteroendocrine cells in the stomach lining, stimulates other gland cells as well as smooth muscle fibers in the stomach wall?

- A) gastrin
- B) cholecystokinin
- C) intrinsic factor
- D) secretin

13

The digestive fluids that mix with chyme in the _____ are secreted by _____.

- A) stomach; the liver and pancreas
- B) biliary apparatus; the liver and gallbladder

C)   duodenum; hepatocytes and cells of the pancreatic lobules and ducts

D)   hepatopancreatic ampulla; hepatocytes and cells of the pancreatic islets

14

In the small intestine, the plicae circulares and villi provide

A)   increased surface area for the absorption of nutrient molecules

B)   attachments for mesenteries suspended from the dorsal body wall

C)   initiation of enterogastric reflexes that accelerate digestion

D)   intestinal contractions that churn and swirl the intestinal chyme

15

Dietary lipids and lipid-soluble vitamins too large to enter the bloodstream directly can first enter the _____ by way of _____.

A)   biliary apparatus; the common bile duct

B)   lymphatic system; lacteals

C)   villi; canaliculi

D)   common hepatic duct; cystic duct

16

The mucosa of the _____ is equipped with abundant, pea-sized or larger _____ that help to protect it from encroaching bacteria.

A)   liver; hepatic sinusoids

B)   jejunum; lymphatic nodules

C)   ileum; Peyer patches

D)   appendix; lymph nodes

17

The hormones produced by the enteroendocrine cells of the intestinal glands include

A)   pepsinogen and gastrin

B)   secretin and cholecystokinin

C)   enterokinase and aminopeptidase

D)   biliverdin and bilirubin

18

The _____ reflex stimulates powerful, peristaltic-like contractions of the teniae coli that produce _____, often during or just after a meal.

  A)   gastroileal; haustral churning
  B)   gastrocolic; mass movements
  C)   deglutition; segmentation
  D)   gag; retching

19

Which ligament of the liver is the remnant of the fetal umbilical vein?

  A)   falciform ligament
  B)   ligamentum teres
  C)   coronary ligament
  D)   ligamentum venosum

20

Between the skeletal and digestive systems, there are three types of _____: one in osteons, one in _____, and one within parietal cells of the gastric glands.

  A)   calcium compounds; hepatic lobules
  B)   calcium compounds; spongy bone
  C)   canaliculi; hepatic lobules
  D)   canaliculi; spongy bone

21

Exocrine secretion by the pancreas is

  A)   stimulated by the hormones cholecystokinin and secretin
  B)   stimulated by parasympathetic activity via the vagus nerve
  C)   inhibited by activity of the sympathetic division of the ANS
  D)   all of the above

22

Where does most nutrient absorption occur?

  A)   in the body of the stomach

B)   in the duodenum

C)   in the jejunum

D)   in the ileum and cecum

23

In the adult, the only remnants of the embryonic ventral mesentery are the

A)   greater omentum and mesentery proper

B)   ligamentum venosum and round ligament of the liver

C)   mesocolon and coronary ligament

D)   lesser omentum and falciform ligament

24

What is the most likely cause of pernicious anemia (a chronic, progressive anemia of older adults), given that it can be successfully treated by administration of vitamin B12?

A)   chronic pancreatitis or gastroenteritis

B)   defective parietal cells in the gastric glands

C)   hemorrhage anywhere in the GI tract submucosa

D)   inadequate dietary intake of iron compounds

25

What do all of the popular medications for reflux esophagitis ("heartburn") and gastroesophageal reflux disease have in common?

A)   they are all carcinogenic if taken for prolonged periods

B)   none is particularly effective at relieving symptoms in most patients

C)   all work by reducing stomach acidity rather than preventing reflux

D)   all of the above

ANSWERS

1. A	5. A	9. A
2. B	6. B	10. C
3. B	7. A	11. D
4. C	8. D	12. A

13. C	18. B	23. D
14. A	19. B	24. B
15. B	20. C	25. C
16. C	21. D	
17. B	22. C	

QUIZ 3

1. A complete living thing, including animals and plants, is called

A) an organism

B) tissue

C) a cell

D) a body system

2. The smallest unit of an organism that can carry out the basic functions of life is

A) an organism

B) tissue

C) an organ

D) a cell

3. A group of similar cells that work together to carry out a specific function is

A) tissue

B) a cell

C) an organism

D) an organ

4. A group of different tissues that work together to perform a specific function is

A) a body system

B) a cell

C) an organ

D) an organism

5. A group of organs that work together to perform a specific function is

A) a cell

B) a body system

C) tissue

D) an organism

6. The teeth and stomach breaking down food into smaller pieces are examples of

A) Mechanical Digestion

B) Chemical Digestion

7. Amylase and Pepsin breaking down starch and proteins are examples of

A) Chemical Digestion

B) Mechanical Digestion

8. A digestive enzyme that breaks down starch. It is found in saliva.

A) Lugol

B) Gastric Juice

C) Amylase

D) Pepsin

9. This carbohydrate begins chemical digestion in the mouth

A) sugar

B) starch

C) fiber

D) fat

10. This muscle helps move food to the back of the mouth for swallowing

A) saliva glands

B) tongue

C) teeth

D) lips

11. This organ prevents food and/or drink from entering the trachea

A) Pyloric Sphincter

B) Tonsils

C) Epiglottis

D) Cardiac Sphincter

12. A moist ball made up of chewed up food and saliva

A) peristalsis

B) chyme

C) bolus

D) gastric juice

13. Regular muscular contractions that move food through the digestive tract.

A) chyme

B) pepsin

C) peristalsis

D) bolus

14. A yellow-brown indicator that turns blue-black when it comes in contact with starch.

A) Amylase Solution

B) Lugol Solution

C) Pepsin Solution

D) Benedict's Solution

15. A chemical indicator that, when added to a solution and heated, changes from blue to light green to red in the presence of increasing concentrations of sugar.

A) Pepsin Solution

B) Amylase Solution

C) Lugol Solution

D) Benedict's Solution

16. One of the three basic food types; needed for building and repair of tissue in the body. Found in beef, egg whites, nuts, and pork.

A) sugar

B) fiber

C) protein

D) starch

17. A pulpy mixture of food and gastric juices. Produced in the stomach, from which it passes into the small intestine.

A) peristalsis

B) amylase

C) bolus

D) chyme

18. A small hole in the lining of the stomach, caused in spots where there is no mucus and the gastric juice begins to digest the stomach wall is called

A) heartburn

B) an ulcer

C) peristalsis

D) chyme

19. The sphincter between the stomach and the small intestine is the

A) Cardiac Sphincter

B) Esophageal Sphincter

C) Epiglottis Sphincter

D) Pyloric Sphincter

20. One of the three basic food types. May be in the form of starch, sugar, or fiber. Found in cereals, breads, and vegetables.

A) carbohydrates

B) proteins

C) minerals

D) fat

21. A protein that is capable of speeding up a chemical reaction.

A) fat

B) fiber

C) enzyme

D) vitamins

22. One of the three basic food types; found in oils and some dairy products.

A) protein

B) carbohydrates

C) fats

D) fiber

23. An indigestible carbohydrate such as cellulose that stimulates peristalsis in the intestine.

A) fiber

B) vitamins

C) fats

D) protein

24. A liquid that includes hydrochloric acid and pepsin and that is responsible for the chemical digestion of protein in the stomach.

A) gastric juice

B) Benedicts

C) vitamins

D) Lugols

25. A painful sensation in the lower esophagus or upper stomach; sometimes caused by excess stomach acid.

A) fiber

B) carbohydrates

C) heartburn

D) vitamins

26. A component of gastric juice that helps create the environment that pepsin needs to break down protein in the stomach.

A) Lugols

B) vitamins

C) Benedicts

D) hydrochloric acid

27. A substance that changes in some way to indicate the presence of another substance. Examples include Benedict's solution and Lugol solution.

A) indicator

B) fiber

C) vitamin

D) mineral

28. An enzyme in the stomach that breaks down protein.

A) benedicts

B) lugols

C) amylase

D) pepsin

29. Watery substance secreted by three pairs of glands around the mouth. Helps moisten and soften food for swallowing.

A) saliva

B) lugols

C) vitamins

D) benedicts

30. The sphincter between the esophagus and the stomach is the

A) Epiglottis Sphincter

B) Esophageal Sphincter

C) Pyloric Sphincter

D) Rectal Sphincter

ANSWERS

1. A 2.D 3.A 4.C 5.B 6.A 7.A 8.C 9.B 10.B 11.C 12.C 13.C 14.B 15.D 16.C 17.D 18.B 19.D 20.A 21.C 22.C 23.A 24.A 25.C 26.D 27.A 28.D 29.A 30.B

QUIZ 4

1. The two organs that produce digestive fluids that are secreted into the small intestine are

A) liver and pancreas

B) gall bladder and jejunum

C) liver and gall bladder

D) colon and gall bladder

2. The tiny projections that cover the surface of the folds in the small intestine are

A) ulcers

B) teeth

C) muscles

D) villi and microvilli

3. The process by which the nutrients from the digested food pass into the blood vessels through the wall of the small intestine is called

A) elimination

B) digestion

C) evaporation

D) diffusion

4. Fats get chemically digested into

A) fatty acids and glycerol

B) bile

C) amino acids and proteins

D) glucose and starch

5. The liquid that breaks down large fat droplets into smaller ones so they can mix more easily with the juices from the small intestine and pancreas is

A) mucus

B) chyme

C) water

D) bile

6. The nutrient(s) that is/are chemically digested in the small intestine are:

A) carbohydrates only

B) carbohydrates, proteins and fats

C) fats only

D) protein only

E) carbohydrates and fats

7. The result of chemically digesting proteins are:

A) carbohydrates

B) amino acids

C) simple sugars

D) bile

8. The result of chemically digesting carbohydrates are

A) amino acids

B) bile

C) carbohydrates

D) simple sugars

9. This material passes through the colon and is composed of water, undigested food, mucus, dead cells, and bacteria.

A) mucus

B) chyme

C) bolus

D) feces

10. This happens when the feces move through the large intestine too quickly and there's not enough time for water to be absorbed (too much water in the feces).

A) diarrhea

B) constipation

C) appendicitis

D) ulcer

11. This happens when the feces move through the colon too slowly and too much water is absorbed (not enough water in the feces).

A) constipation

B) nausea

C) diarrhea

D) vomiting

12. These pass through the walls of the large intestine into the bloodstream.

A) bile and chyme

B) enzymes

C) water and minerals

D) nutrients

13. The substance produced by the liver is

A) pepsin

B) amylase

C) bile

D) renin

14. A liquid that is basic/alkaline (not acidic) and is used to neutralize stomach acid.

A) gastric juice

B) bile

C) mucus

D) pancreatic juice

Quest

15. Diffusion is often called passive transport because

A) It takes place only in water

B) Energy from the cell IS needed for it to occur

C) Energy from the cell is NOT needed for it to occur

D) It takes place only without water

16. When the appendix gets blocked, it becomes swollen and infected by bacteria. This condition is called?

A) ulcer

B) heartburn

C) constipation

D) appendicitis

17. A medication that causes the peristaltic contractions (squeezing) to increase and to move wastes through the large intestine more quickly.

A) antacid

B) laxative

C) vitamin

D) mineral

18. This is released when bacteria in the large intestine start to feast on undigested food.

A) water

B) mucus

C) gas

D) acid

ANSWERS

1. A 2.D 3.D 4.A 5.D 6.B 7.B 8.D 9.D 10.A 11.A 12.C 13.C 14.D 15.C 16.D 17.B 18.C

QUIZ 5

1. The enzyme found in saliva is

A) Pepsin

B) Amylase

C) Lugol

D) Gastric Juice

2. This carbohydrate begins digestion in the mouth

A) fat

B) sugar

C) starch

D) fiber

3. This organ prevents food and/or drink from entering the trachea (wind pipe)

A) Cardiac Sphincter

B) Epiglottis

C) Tonsils

D) Pyloric Sphincter

4. When food is chewed and mixed with saliva, it turns into a moist ball or

A) bolus

B) gastric juice

C) chyme

D) peristalsis

5. The wavelike muscle contractions that move food down the esophagus is called

A) pepsin

B) bolus

C) chyme

D) peristalsis

6. This indicator solution is used to test for starch

A) Pepsin Solution

B) Benedict's Solution

C) Amylase Solution

D) Lugol Solution

7. This indicator solution is used to test for sugar

A) Benedict's Solution

B) Pepsin Solution

C) Amylase Solution

D) Lugol Solution

8. Gastric juices start the digestion of

A) protein

B) fiber

C) starch

D) sugar

9. The pulpy mixture of food and gastric juices in the stomach is called

A) peristalsis

B) bolus

C) chyme

D) amylase

10. A small hole in the lining of the stomach, caused in spots where there is no mucus and the gastric juice begins to digest the stomach wall is called

A) peristalsis

B) chyme

C) heartburn

D) an ulcer

11. The sphincter between the stomach and the small intestine is the

A) Cardiac Sphincter

B) Epiglottis Sphincter

C) Pyloric Sphincter

D) Esophagus Sphincter

12. The first 25cm of the small intestine is called the

A) colon

B) duodenum

C) jejunum

D) ileum

13. The two organs that produce digestive fluids that are secreted into the small intestine are

A) gall bladder and jejunum

B) liver and gall bladder

C) liver and pancreas

D) colon and gall bladder

14. The tiny projections that cover the surface of the folds in the small intestine are

A) ulcers

B) teeth

C) muscles

D) villi and microvilli

15. The process by which the nutrients from the digested food pass into the blood vessels through the wall of the small intestine is called

A) diffusion

B) digestion

C) elimination

D) evaporation

16. The three parts of the small intestine are the duodenum, jejunum and ileum?

A) True

B) False

17. Fats get chemically digested into

A) glucose and starch

B) amino acids and proteins

C) fatty acids and glycerol

D) bile

18. The liquid that breaks down large fat droplets into smaller ones so they can mix more easily with the juices from the small intestine and pancreas is

A) chyme

B) mucus

C) water

D) bile

19. The nutrient(s) that is/are chemically digested in the small intestine are:

A) carbohydrates, proteins and fats

B) fats only

C) protein only

D) carbohydrates only

E) carbohydrates and fats

20. The result of chemically digesting proteins are:

A) amino acids

B) simple sugars

C) carbohydrates

D) bile

21. The result of chemically digesting carbohydrates are

A) bile

B) amino acids

C) carbohydrates

D) simple sugars

22. This organ was once used to help digest the cellulose in plant matter, but it is not useful now. It needs to be surgically removed if it becomes infected by bacteria.

A) gall bladder

B) liver

C) appendix

D) pancreas

23. This material passes through the colon and is composed of water, undigested food, mucus, dead cells, and bacteria.

A) feces

B) chyme

C) bolus

D) mucus

24. When the feces move through the large intestine too quickly and there's not enough time for water to be absorbed (too much water in the feces).

A) constipation

B) ulcer

C) diarrhea

D) appendicitis

25. When the feces move through the colon too slowly and too much water is absorbed (not enough water in the feces).

A) vomiting

B) nausea

C) constipation

D) diarrhea

26. These pass through the walls of the large intestine into the bloodstream.

A) nutrients

B) enzymes

C) water and minerals

D) bile and chyme

27. The organ that stores bile and pumps it into the duodenum is:

A) colon

B) appendix

C) pancreas

D) gall bladder

28. The substance produced by the liver is

A) pepsin

B) amylase

C) renin

D) bile

29. The largest internal organ is:

A) gall bladder

B) heart

C) stomach

D) liver

30. A liquid that is basic/alkaline (not acidic) and is used to neutralize stomach acid.

A) bile

B) mucus

C) pancreatic juice

D) gastric juice

31. The amount of juice secreted by the pancreas secretes every day.

A) .05 liters

B) 1.5 liters

C) 10 liters

D) 100 liters

ANSWERS

1. B 2.C 3.B 4.A 5.D 6.D 7.A 8.A 9.C 10.D 11.C 12.B 13.C 14.D 15.A
16.A 17.C 18.D 19.A 20.A 21.D 22.C 23.A 24.C 25.C 26.C 27.D 28.D
29.D 30.C 31.B

MUSCULAR SYSTEM

QUIZ 1

1

The layer of connective tissue that separates the muscle tissue into small sections is called the
_____.
- A) aponeuroses
- B) epimysium
- C) perimysium
- D) endomysium

2

The segment of a myofibril that is called a sarcomere runs from _____.
- A) one Z line to the next Z line
- B) one H zone to the next H zone
- C) one A band to the next A band
- D) one end of a skeletal muscle to the opposite end

3

The _____ are an invagination of the muscle cell's sarcolemma.
- A) sarcoplasmic reticula
- B) transverse (T) tubules
- C) cisternae
- D) microtubules

4

Into what does the neuron release its neurotransmitter at the neuromuscular junction?
- A) motor end plate
- B) cytoplasm of the muscle cell
- C) cisternae
- D) synaptic cleft

5

A motor unit is made up of _____.

A) all the muscle fibers within a given muscle
B) a motor neuron and the muscle fibers it innervates
C) all the neurons going into an individual section of the body
D) a fascicle and a nerve

6

The cross bridges involved in muscle contraction are located on the _____ .
A) myosin myofilaments
B) actin myofilaments
C) tropomyosin
D) dystrophin

7

Which of these statements is correct regarding muscle contraction?
A) All motor units act together.
B) Muscle contraction continues for long periods after nervous stimulation ceases.
C) The cross bridges bind to the actin and shorten the sarcomeres.
D) Dystrophin is not needed to strengthen the contracting muscle cell.

8

When a nervous impulse travels from a neuron to a muscle cell, what happens next?
A) The impulse travels over the sarcolemma in all directions.
B) Calcium is released from the sarcoplasmic reticulum.
C) Linkages form between the actin and myosin.
D) Acetylcholine is decomposed by acetylcholinesterase.

9

One of the following statements about muscular responses is not true. Choose that one.
A) A muscle fiber contracts in an all-or-none fashion.
B) There is a slight latent period that occurs between when the stimulus arrives at the muscle and when the muscle contracts.
C) Muscles will add motor units to a contraction, increasing the overall force of contraction.
D) When a person is fully at rest, none of her muscles are contracting.

10

The type of muscle found in the irises of the eyes and in the blood vessels is called
_____.

A) visceral smooth muscle
B) multiunit smooth muscle
C) cardiac muscle
D) skeletal muscle

11

Why can cardiac muscle fibers contract for longer periods than skeletal muscle fibers?

A) Cardiac muscle is self-excitatory.
B) Extracellular calcium partially controls the strength (and length) of contraction.
C) Cisternae of T-tubules is more developed in cardiac muscle.
D) Cardiac muscle is uninucleate rather than multinucleate.

12

Which muscle enables you to pucker your lips for a kiss?

A) epicranius
B) buccinator
C) orbicularis oris
D) orbicularis oculi

13

The muscle that enables you to elevate and adduct your scapula is the _____.

A) serratus anterior
B) sternocleidomastoid
C) splenius capitis
D) rhomboideus major

14

Which muscle is the strongest flexor of the elbow?

A) brachialis
B) biceps brachii
C) brachioradialis
D) deltoid

15

The biceps femoris is one hamstring muscle located on the back of the thigh. Which muscle is the other hamstring?
- A)   adductor magnus
- B)   semitendinosus
- C)   gluteus maximus
- D)   quadriceps femoris

16

Which of the following does not belong with the others?
- A)   multinucleated
- B)   skeletal
- C)   striated
- D)   involuntary

17

Each muscle fiber is directly surrounded by connective tissue called the _____.
- A)   perimysium
- B)   fascia
- C)   endomysium
- D)   epimysium

18

Which term is the smallest subdivision in this group?
- A)   fiber
- B)   fibril
- C)   filament
- D)   actin

19

Which description of muscle contraction means that all of the fibers within a muscle are fully contracted?
- A)   all-or-none law
- B)   summation
- C)   tetanic
- D)   muscle twitching

20

The application of multiple stimuli to a muscle is defined as the process called _____.
- A) tetany
- B) summation
- C) fatigue
- D) treppe

21

The term _____ refers to the constant state of contraction of a certain number of fibers within a muscle.
- A) atrophy
- B) hypertrophy
- C) summation
- D) tone

22

Muscles that are not used may degenerate or undergo a process of _____.
- A) atrophy
- B) hypertrophy
- C) fatigue
- D) tetany

23

Muscles that act to cause similar movements are called _____.
- A) antagonists
- B) origins
- C) insertions
- D) synergists

24

The major muscle lining the cheek is the _____.
- A) orbicularis oculi
- B) orbicularis oris
- C) zygomaticus

D) buccinator

25

The triangle shaped muscle which antagonizes the sternocleidomastoid is the _____.
    A) deltoid
    B) pectoralis major
    C) external oblique
    D) trapezius

26

The antagonist to the triceps brachii is the _____.
    A) deltoid
    B) pectoralis major
    C) brachialis
    D) serratus anterior

ANSWERS

1. C
2. A
3. B
4. D
5. B
6. A
7. C
8. A
9. D
10. B
11. B
12. C
13. D
14. A
15. B
16. D
17. C
18. D
19. C
20. B
21. D
22. A
23. D

24. D
25. D
26. C

QUIZ 2

1

Which of the following types of muscle are found in the stomach or blood vessels?

    A)   cardiac
    B)   skeletal
    C)   visceral
    D)   striated

2

A large broad sheet of connective tissue, such as on the abdomen, is called a/an _____ .

    A)   aponeurosis
    B)   epimysium
    C)   perimysium
    D)   endomysium

3

The membrane that is the closest to the individual muscle fiber is the _____ .

    A)   aponeurosis
    B)   epimysium
    C)   perimysium
    D)   endomysium

4

A group of skeletal muscle fibers is called a/an _____ .

    A)   perimysium
    B)   fascicle
    C)   epimysium
    D)   tendon

5

The structure that connects muscles to bones is the _____ .

A) aponeurosis
B) fascicle
C) tendon
D) ligament

6

The fibers of a muscle that are connected to the overlying skin fibers is the _____ .
A) subcutaneous fascia
B) deep fascia
C) subserous fascia
D) tendon

7

The muscle cells within a group such as the biceps brachii are individually called _____ .
A) sarcolemmas
B) fibers
C) myocyte
D) myofibrils

8

The fiber cell membrane is termed the _____ .
A) myofibril
B) myosin
C) myofilament
D) sarcolemma

9

Which of the following does not belong with the others?
A) myofilament
B) myosin
C) myofibril
D) actin

10

The smallest, functional unit of contraction is the _____ .

A)   fiber
B)   sarcomere
C)   filament
D)   myofibril

11

The I bands in a sarcomere are made of _____ .
    A)   myosin
    B)   actin and myosin
    C)   tropomyosin
    D)   actin

12

The _____ zone contains only myosin and is in the center of a sarcomere.
    A)   A
    B)   I
    C)   M
    D)   H

13

The cisternae are enlarged portions of the _____ .
    A)   sarcoplasmic reticulum
    B)   endoplasmic reticulum
    C)   transverse tubules
    D)   T-tubules

14

The gap between the muscle and a nerve is the _____ .
    A)   synapse
    B)   motor end plate
    C)   myoneural junction
    D)   motor neuron

15

The chemical that crosses a neuromuscular gap is _____ .

A) sodium
B) a protein
C) a neurotransmitter
D) calcium

16

The combination of a neuron and the muscle fiber it associates with is called a/an _____ .
A)   fascicle
B)   motor end plate
C)   motor unit
D)   myoneural junction

17

The most abundant of the muscle proteins is _____ .
A)   actin
B)   troponin
C)   myosin
D)   tropomyosin

18

The main force of contraction occurs when actin forms a chemical complex with _____ .
A)   troponin
B)   myosin
C)   tropomyosin
D)   acetylcholine

19

When a muscle is at rest, which of the following is not associated chemically with the others?
A)   actin
B)   myosin
C)   troponin
D)   tropomyosin

20

During the contraction of a sarcomere, calcium ions bind with the protein _____ .

A)   actin
B)   myosin
C)   troponin
D)   tropomyosin

21

The main neurotransmitter involved in skeletal muscle contraction is _____.
A)   adrenalin
B)   noradrenalin
C)   acetylcholine
D)   dopamine

22

Which molecule directly supplies energy to myosin to allow the filaments to contract?
A)   adenosine diphosphate
B)   ATP
C)   creatine phosphate
D)   creatinine

23

What is the most abundant storage form of energy within a muscle fiber?
A)   glycogen
B)   ADP
C)   ATP
D)   creatine phosphate

24

What effect does creatine phosphokinase have an muscle activity?
A)   it causes a fiber to relax
B)   it stimulates ATP synthesis
C)   catalyzes the formation of creatine phosphate
D)   causes the breakdown or creatine into creatinine

25

How is excess sugar stored within muscle fibers?

A) in ATP
B) glycogen
C) glucose
D) creatinine

26

Which main factor allows muscle to sustain contraction even during times when the blood supply is low?
A) the presence of hemoglobin
B) glycogen storage
C) myoglobin
D) citric acid cycle

27

The reddish brown color of muscle is due to the presence of _____ molecules.
A) creatine phosphate
B) hemoglobin
C) iron
D) myoglobin

28

Which molecule is produced during exercise, resulting in the oxygen debt?
A) glycogen
B) lactate
C) pyruvate
D) ATP

29

Which of the following does not belong with the others?
A) white muscles
B) fast-contracting
C) extensive sarcoplasmic reticulum
D) relatively large supply of myoglobin

30

About _____% of ATP energy becomes liberated as heat from muscle metabolism.
  A)   25
  B)   50
  C)   75
  D)   10

31

The minimum stimulus needed to cause a contraction is called the _____.
  A)   all-or-none law
  B)   threshold
  C)   sub-maximal stimulus
  D)   recruitment level

32

A single contraction of a muscle is called a _____.
  A)   threshold
  B)   recruitment
  C)   twitch
  D)   myogram

33

The period of time between the stimulus and contraction is called the _____.
  A)   latent period
  B)   refractory period
  C)   contraction period
  D)   relaxation period

34

The period of time in which a muscle will not respond to a stimulus is called the _____.
  A)   latent period
  B)   refractory period
  C)   relaxation period
  D)   threshold

35

The complete contraction of a muscle, without the ability to relax, is called _____.
- A) a sustained contraction
- B) fatigue
- C) tetanic contraction
- D) treppe

36

The constant contraction of a percentage of fibers within a muscle is referred to as _____.
- A) tetany
- B) tonus
- C) sustained contraction
- D) summation

37

Contractions called _____ occur whenever the forces applied to a muscle are increased, but the muscle does not appear to be moving.
- A) isotonic
- B) isometric
- C) tetanic
- D) summation contractions

38

Which of the following muscles always requires nerve impulses in order to contract?
- A) multi-unit smooth
- B) skeletal
- C) visceral smooth
- D) cardiac

39

Which type of muscle is found in the wall of blood vessels?
- A) skeletal
- B) cardiac
- C) smooth visceral
- D) multi-unit smooth

40

Since smooth muscle fibers have rhythmicity and can stimulate each other, they contract in a pattern called _____.
- A) a functional syncytium
- B) peristalsis
- C) tetany
- D) tonus

41

The degeneration of muscle fibers caused by a lack of proper stimulation and usage is called
_____.
- A) hypertrophy
- B) atrophy
- C) dystrophy
- D) peristalsis

42

In smooth muscle, calcium ions combine with _____ to allow the actin and myosin cross-bridges to form.
- A) calmodulin
- B) troponin
- C) myosin
- D) tropomyosin

43

The following cause smooth muscles to contract except which one?
- A) acetylcholine
- B) troponin
- C) norepinephrine
- D) oxytocin

44

The presence of _____ allow cardiac muscle fibers to transmit impulses faster among themselves.
- A) cell membranes
- B) nerve fibers
- C) intercalated disks

D)   peristalsis

45

The muscle is called the _____ when it is causing the movement that is being described.
A)   antagonist
B)   synergist
C)   prime mover
D)   flexor

46

Muscles that act together to cause the same movements are called _____.
A)   synergists
B)   antagonists
C)   prime movers
D)   agonists

47

The sternocleidomastoid muscle was named because of its _____.
A)   shape
B)   size
C)   location
D)   points of attachment

48

The _____ muscle forms a broad flat sheet on top of the head.
A)   temporalis
B)   buccinator
C)   epicranius
D)   frontalis

49

Which muscle lines most of the inner cheek wall?
A)   orbicularis oris
B)   buccinator
C)   orbicularis oculi

D) masseter

50

Which muscle causes smiling and is attached to the corners of the lips?
    A)   zygomatic
    B)   buccinator
    C)   temporalis
    D)   orbicularis oris

ANSWERS

1. C	33. A
2. A	34. B
3. D	35. C
4. B	36. B
5. C	37. B
6. B	38. B
7. B	39. D
8. D	40. B
9. C	41. B
10. B	42. A
11. D	43. B
12. D	44. C
13. A	45. C
14. C	46. A
15. C	47. D
16. C	48. C
17. C	49. B
18. B	50. A
19. B	
20. C	
21. C	
22. B	
23. D	
24. C	
25. B	
26. C	
27. D	
28. B	
29. D	
30. C	
31. B	
32. D	

QUIZ 3

1) _____ occurs when body temperature falls below normal levels.

    A.   Hyperthermia (Your Answer)
    B.   Hypothermia (Correct Answer)
    C.   Chills

2)   Muscular tissue produces body movement; stabilizes body position, regulates organ volume, moves substances within the body and produces heat

    A.   True
    B.   False

3)   What striated muscle tissue is attached to bones and moving parts of the skeleton?

    A.   Connective tissue
    B.   Smooth tissue
    C.   Skeletal tissue

4)   Muscle contraction that produces movement of a joint.

    A.   Isotonic
    B.   Isometric
    C.   Abduction
    D.   Adduction

5) _____ muscle contractions don't always produce movement

    A.   Isometric
    B.   Isotonic
    C.   Tetanic

6)
True or false: Tonic Contraction move body parts and hold muscles in position.

    A.   True
    B.   False

7)   Smooth muscle tissue is:

A. Non striated
B. Voluntary
C. Involuntary
D. Striated
E. Both A &C

8) Muscles move bones by _____ on them.

A. Pushing
B. Pulling

9) Is ATP used or produced by muscle?

A. Produced
B. Used

10) These are striated muscles

A. Skeletal
B. Cardiac
C. Smooth
D. A&B
E. B&C

11) What kind of muscle contraction would help a person with hypothermia?

12) When bending the elbow, the origin is at the _____

13) A muscle produces ATP

A. True
B. False

14)
Any muscle inflammation is termed

A. Myositis
B. Myoistis
C. Myostisis
D. Myoititis

15) Most skeletal muscle attach to (#)_____ bones and have a moveable _____
Between them.

    A.   1 bone, moveable tendon
    B.   2 bones, moveable joint
    C.   4 bones, moveable ligament

16) A muscle cell are also called _____

17) Lifting something is an example of what kind skeletal muscle contraction?

    A.   Flexion
    B.   Extension
    C.   Isometric Contraction
    D.   Isotonic Contraction

18) If a prime mover caused extension, the antagonist would cause _____

    A.   Rotation
    B.   Flexion
    C.   Isometric contractions

19) A quick jerky response to a stimulus is called a _____

20) The muscles attachment to the more stationary bone.

    A.   Connective tissue
    B.   Origin
    C.   Rotation

21) For muscle contractions to occur, the body needs

    A.   Tendons and joints
    B.   ATP and Calcium
    C.   Mitochondria and X chromosomes
    D.   Sodium and Calcium

22)
enter/o refers to

    A.   Small intestine
    B.   Intestines
    C.   Colon
    D.   Both A & B

23)   When muscles are constantly stimulated and the strength of muscle contractions decrease it is known as

    A.   Oxygen debt
    B.   Fatigue
    C.   Atrophy
    D.   Myalgia

24)   What attach muscle to bones at both origin and insertion sites?

25)   This type of muscle tissue is located in the walls of hallow internal structures such as stomach, blood vessels, and air ways

    A.   Skeletal muscle tissue
    B.   Smooth muscle tissue
    C.   Cardiac muscle tissue
    D.   Both A&C

26)   _____ _____ _____ is an autoimmune muscle disorder.

27)
Muscular dystrophy is a chronic disease characterized by muscle weakness.

    A.   True
    B.   False

28)   _____ anchor muscle firmly to bones

29) Tendon Sheaths and bursae perform this function

    A.   Attaching muscle to bone
    B.   Temperature regulation
    C.   Lubrication

30) The muscles _____ is its attachment to the to the more moveable bone

    A.   Insertion
    B.   Extension

31) This type of contraction is responsible for maintaining posture

    A.   Tetanic contraction
    B.   Tonic contraction
    C.   Isometric contraction

32) Muscle contractions causing shivering would produce _____

ANSWERS

1. B
2. A
3. C
4. A
5. A
6. B
7. E
8. B
9. B
10. D
11. SHIVERING
12. SHOULDER
13. B
14. A
15. B
16. MUSCLE FIBERS
17. D

18. B
19. TWITCH
20. B
21. B
22. D
23. B
24. TENDON
25. B
26. DUCHENNE'S MUSCULAR DYSTROPHY
27. B
28. TENDONS
29. C
30. A
31. B
32. HEAT

SKELETAL SYSTEM

1

Which of the following account(s) for the variance in the number of bones?

A)   age
B)   genetic variation
C)   sex
D)   both a and b

2

Bones that form in tendons in response to stress are called

A)   cartilaginous bones
B)   sesamoid bones
C)   latent bones
D)   spongy bones

3

Which of the following is (are) not a part of the axial skeleton?

A)   auditory ossicles
B)   ribs
C)   os coxae
D)   both b and c

4

Which of the following is not a part of the appendicular skeleton?

    A)   the vertebral column
    B)   the patella
    C)   the clavicle
    D)   the femur

5

Which of the following is not a function of the skeletal system?
    A)   support
    B)   hemopoiesis
    C)   mineral storage
    D)   coordination

6

Which of the following is (are) not protected by the skeletal system?
    A)   liver
    B)   heart
    C)   muscles
    D)   central nervous system

7

Bone is primarily composed of
    A)   phosphorous
    B)   calcium
    C)   magnesium
    D)   both a and b

8

In function, the skeletal system is most closely associated with the
    A)   muscular system
    B)   mineral system
    C)   nervous system
    D)   urinary system

9

Which of the following is not one of the categories of bone shape?
- A) long bones
- B) flat bones
- C) thick bones
- D) short bones

10

The type of bone that most commonly functions as a lever is
- A) irregular bone
- B) thick bone
- C) long bone
- D) short bone
- E) sesamoid bone

11

A facet is described as a (136)
- A) marked bony prominence
- B) sharp, slender process
- C) flattened or shallow articulating surface
- D) projection adjacent to a condyle

12

A small pit or depression on a bone is referred to as a (136)
- A) fossa
- B) fissure
- C) fovea
- D) meatus

13

Red bone marrow within certain long bones is in contact with the (137)
- A) articular cartilage
- B) endosteum
- C) epiphyseal plate
- D) periosteum

14

Large bone cells that enzymatically break down bone tissue and that play an important role in bone growth, remodeling, and healing are known as (138)
    A)   osteogenic cells
    B)   osteoblasts
    C)   osteocytes
    D)   osteoclasts
    E)   bone-lining cells

15

The bone cells that are thought to regulate the movement of calcium and phosphate into and out of bone matrix are known as (138)
    A)   osteogenic cells
    B)   osteoblasts
    C)   osteocytes
    D)   osteoclasts
    E)   bone-lining cells

16

Osteocytes within compact bone tissue are located in minute capsules, or spaces, known as (138)
    A)   lacunae
    B)   osteons
    C)   lamellae
    D)   trabeculae
    E)   sinuses

17

In compact bone, the matrix is laid down in concentric rings called (140)
    A)   osteons
    B)   lamellae
    C)   canaliculi
    D)   trabeculae
    E)   osteons

18

_____ builds up bone, while _____ breaks down bone. (138)

A) Meatus/marrow
B) Osteoblast activity/osteoclast activity
C) Epiphysis/diaphysis
D) Diaphysis/epiphysis

19

Calcification is the process of (140)
A) ossification
B) osteoporosis
C) growth
D) mitosis

20

_____ is the process by which minerals are deposited in the matrix of cartilaginous bone tissue. (140)
A) Ossification
B) Hardening
C) Calcification
D) Deposition

21

Spongy bone develops at the _____ _____ centers. (142)
A) bone marrow
B) histological zone
C) primary ossification
D) secondary ossification

22

A(n) _____ _____ consists of five histological zones. (142)
A) Epiphyseal plate
B) primary ossification center
C) secondary ossification center
D) cartilage ring

23

The _____ is a region of transformation from cartilage tissue to bone tissue. (143)
- A) ossification zone
- B) calcification zone
- C) cartilage ring
- D) none of the above

24

The fontanels permit (144)
- A) rapid growth of the brain
- B) passage of heat
- C) molding during parturition
- D) both a and c

25

Which is not one of the six fontanels? (144)
- A) lateral fontanel
- B) posterior fontanel
- C) anterior fontanel
- D) all of these are fontanels

26

Which is not a bone forming the orbit? (151)
- A) frontal bone
- B) zygomatic bone
- C) maxilla
- D) occipital bone

27

The mastoid process is a bony extension of the (151)
- A) occipital bone
- B) parietal bone
- C) sphenoid bone
- D) zygomatic bone
- E) temporal bone

28

The sella turcica, supporting the pituitary gland, is part of the (152)

  A)   frontal bone
  B)   sphenoid bone
  C)   nasal bone
  D)   ethmoid bone

29

Which statement explains why facial bones are not classified as cranial bones? (154)

  A)   Facial bones do not come in contact with the brain.
  B)   They are lighter in weight than cranial bones.
  C)   The cranial bones have cavities.
  D)   None of the above.

30

Which is not a facial bone? (154)

  A)   zygomatic bone
  B)   lacrimal bone
  C)   vomer
  D)   all of these are facial bones

31

The functions of the vertebral column do not include (159)

  A)   protection of the spinal cord
  B)   support for the head
  C)   attachment site for muscles
  D)   reflex action

32

Which of the following is not one of the four curvatures of the vertebral column? (159)

  A)   brachial curve
  B)   thoracic curve
  C)   cervical curve
  D)   lumbar curve

33

Processes that limit the twisting of the vertebral column are the (160)

A) spinous processes
B) transverse processes
C) lateral processes
D) articular processes

34

A structural feature of a typical cervical vertebra is (160)

A) transverse foramen
B) a dens
C) a long spinous process
D) a fovea

35

Which of the following is (are) not considered part of the rib cage? (164)

A) clavicles
B) false ribs
C) sternum
D) costal cartilages

36

The three components of the sternum, listed from superior to inferior in position, are (164)

A) xiphoid process, sternal angle, costal notch
B) manubrium, body, xiphoid process
C) jugular notch, clavicular notch, costal notch
D) body, manubrium, clavicular notch

37

Which portion of the sternum attaches to the greatest number of ribs? (164)

A) manubrium
B) body
C) xiphoid process
D) all attach to the same number

38

Certain structures are common to all ribs; for example, a (165)

A) tubercle
B) head
C) neck
D) both b and c

39

An abnormal condition in a child due to a lack of vitamin D is (166)

A) osteomalacia
B) rickets
C) acromegaly
D) gigantism

40

Osteoporosis, the disorder characterized by weakening of bones, primarily as a result of calcium loss, is most common in which group? (167)

A) postmenopausal women
B) elderly men
C) children
D) all adults

41

Hypersecretion of the pituitary growth hormone in an adult may result in (166)

A) Paget's disease
B) osteoporosis
C) acromegaly
D) osteomalacia

42

The most virulent type of bone cancer, which frequently metastasizes through the blood to the lungs, is (167)

A) osteoid osteomas
B) osteoma
C) osteogenic sarcoma
D) none; bone cancer is not virulent

43

A fissure is defined as (136)
    A)   a deep pit or socket
    B)   a rounded opening through a bone
    C)   a groove that accommodates a vessel, nerve, or tendon
    D)   a narrow, slitlike opening

44

Which of the following is found only on the femur? (136)
    A)   tubercle
    B)   trochanter
    C)   tuberosity
    D)   head

45

Which of the following is found only on the humerus?
    A)   tubercle
    B)   trochanter
    C)   tuberosity
    D)   head

46

Which of the following associations is not correct? (137)
    A)   endosteum/yellow bone marrow
    B)   medullary cavity/endosteum
    C)   medullary cavity/periosteum
    D)   red bone marrow/spongy bone

47

Which of the following secures the periosteum to the bone? (137)
    A)   perforating fibers
    B)   epiphyseal plate
    C)   endosteum
    D)   diploe

48

Trabeculae (138)
- A)   are found in spongy bone
- B)   give spongy bone a latticework appearance
- C)   are found in compact bone
- D)   both a and b

49

Ossification of the fontanels is normally completed by (144)
- A)   6-12 months
- B)   12-18 months
- C)   18-24 months
- D)   24-30 months

50

Which of the following foramen/structure transmitted associations is not correct? (146)
- A)   carotid canal/internal carotid artery
- B)   foramen ovale/mandibular branch of trigeminal nerve
- C)   foramen rotundum/mandibular branch of trigeminal nerve
- D)   mandibular foramen/inferior alveolar nerve

51

Which is not a sinus found in the skull? (151)
- A)   sphenoidal
- B)   frontal
- C)   ethmoidal
- D)   maxillary
- E)   all of the above are sinuses found in the skull

52

Which of the following is a primary curve of the vertebral column? (159)
- A)   cervical
- B)   lumbar
- C)   thoracic
- D)   pelvic

E)   both c and d

53

Which is not a characteristic of lumbar vertebrae? (161)
     A)   thin, long spinous processes
     B)   transverse foramina
     C)   large bodies
     D)   thick spinous processes
     E)   both a and b

54

Which of the following is not a portion of the developing skull? (141)
     A)   mesocranium
     B)   neurocranium
     C)   chondrocranium
     D)   viscerocranium

ANSWERS

	23. A	46. C
1. D	24. D	47. A
2. B	25. A	48. D
3. C	26. D	49. C
4. A	27. E	50. C
5. D	28. B	51. E
6. C	29. A	52. E
7. D	30. D	53. E
8. A	31. D	54. A
9. C	32. A	
10. C	33. D	
11. C	34. A	
12. C	35. A	
13. B	36. B	
14. D	37. B	
15. E	38. D	
16. A	39. B	
17. B	40. A	
18. B	41. C	
19. A	42. C	
20. C	43. D	
21. D	44. B	
22. A	45. A	

QUIZ 2

1.

Which of the following is not part of axial skeleton?

a) Sternum
b) Mandible
c) Humerus
d) Sacrum
e) Calvarium

2.

All the following are components of appendicular skeleton except

a) Clavicle
b) Femur
c) Pelvic bone
d) Vertebrae
e) Carpal bones

3.

The paraxial mesoderm around the neural tube gives rise to......

a) Scleretome
b) Somites
c) Ectoderm
d) Dermomyotome
e) Neural crest

4.

The bones of the pelvic and shoulder girdles are from the mesenchymal cells form......

a) Paraxial mesoderm
b) Lateral plate mesoderm

c) Intermediate mesoderm
d) General mesoderm
e) Neural crest

5.

During chondrogenesis, the mesenchymal cells first differentiate in to......

a) Osteoblasts
b) Chondrocytes
c) Chondroblasts
d) Chondroclasts
e) None of the above

6.

The organic component of bone matrix is produced by:

a) Osteoblasts
b) Osteocytes
c) Osteoclasts
d) Chondrocytes
e) Chondroblasts

7.

Which of the following cell types is responsible for synthesizing the organic component of cartilage matrix?

a) Osteocytes
b) Chondrocytes
c) Osteoblasts
d) Chodroblasts
e) Chondroclasts

8.

.... are cells that tear down and remodel bone

a) Macrophages
b) Osteocytes
c) Osteocytes
d) Chondroclasts
e) Osteoclasts

9.

Intramembranous and Endochondral are 2 mechanisms of:

a) Tissue deposition
b) Bone remodeling
c) Embryonic skeletal ossification
d) Cartilage resorption
e) None of the above

10.

The flant bones of the skull develop by mean of....

a) Endochondoral ossification
b) Intramembranous ossification
c) Calvarium ossification
d) Internal ossification
e) External ossification

11.

Temporary openings between the cranial bones at birth are:

a) Cranial openings
b) Frontal sinuses
c) Fontanelles
d) Epiphyseal plates
e) Cribifrom plates

12.

After birth, continuous remodelling of bones occurs by coordinate action of...

a) Osteocytes and osteoblasts
b) Osteocytes and osteoclasts
c) Osteoblasts and osteoclats
d) Chondroblast and chondroclasts
e) All of the above

13.

The two sources of membranous neuorocranium are ....

a) Paraxial and lateral mesoderm
b) Paraxial mesoderm and neural crest cells
c) Lateral mesoderm and neural crest cells
d) Ectoderm and endoderm
e) Intermediate mesoderm and neuroectoderm

14.

The mandibular process of the first arch develop in to

a) mandibular process
b) Mandible
c) Maxillae
d) Mandible and maxillae
e) Facial bones

15.

The Mickel's cartilage forms

a) Malleus and incus
b) Incus and stapes
c) Malleus and stapes
d) Ear ossicles
e) Styloid process

16.

The first sets of bones that become fully ossified in the human embryo are

a) Neurocranium
b) Ear ossicles
c) Clavicles and hip bone
d) Viscerocranium
e) Vertebral column

17.

During development, the notochord degenerate and form the....

a) Centrum
b) Nucleus pulposus
c) Annulus fibrose
d) Intervertebral disc
e) Vertebral arch

18.

The outer covering of each bone made from connective tissue is called

a) Perichondrium
b) Periosteum
c) Diaphysis
d) Outer layer
e) External cartilage

19.

.......exacts an inductive influence on the limb mesenchyme to initiate the growth and development of limb bones

a) Apical ectodermal ridge
b) Ectodermal apical ridge
c) Apical mesodermal ridge
d) Apical limb ridge
e) Limbs inductor

20.

The long shaft of the long bone is called

a) Epiphysis
b) Diaphragm
c) Diaphysis
d) Metaphysis
e) Diaphyseal shaft

21.

Growth in the length of the long bone occurs at.....

a)   Periosteum
b)   Diaphysis
c)   Epiphysis
d)   Epiphysial plate
e)   Diaphysial plate

22.

.... is the junction between the diphysis and epiphysis of the growing bone

a)   Articular cartilage
b)   Epiphysial cartilage
c)   Epiphysial plates
d)   Diaphysial-epiphysial junction
e)   Diaphysial plates

For question 23-28, choice whether the statement is True or False

23. The anterior fontanelle closes earlier than the posteror fontanelle

24. At birth, both the diaphysis and epiphysis of long bone are largely ossified

25. The entire limb skeleton is cartilaginous by the end of week six

26. During limb development, the upper limb rotate 90 medially

27. Most of the skeleton in the embryo is cartilage

28. The limb buds become visible as an outpocketings from the dorsomedail body wall

29.

  Excess of pituitary growth hormone will result in a condition called......

a) Cretinism
b) Dwarfism
c) Acromegaly
d) Giantism
e) None of the above

30.

Incomplete closure of the vertebral column results in:

a) Scoliosis
b) Spina bifida
c) Lordosis
d) Kyphosis
e) Vertebral fissure

31.

A letaral deviation of the alignment of the vertebral column is called a

a) Lordosis
b) Kyphosis
c) Scoliosis
d) Lateral deviation
e) Vertebral deviation

32.

Premature closure of the cranial sutures may result to condition known as......

a) Craniosynostosis
b) Acrania
c) Microcephaly
d) Cranioschisis
e) Hydrocephalus

33.

All the following are common types of limb anomalies except

a) Amelia
b) Meromelia
c) Micromelia
d) Phocomelia
e) Sternomelai

34.

..... is type of spina bifida involving the spinal cord and meninges.

a) Spina bifida meninga
b) Spina bifida occulta
c) Spina bifida cystica
d) Spina bifida chordoma
e) Spina bifida vertebrata

35.

..... is a deformity in which the sole of the foot is turned medially and the foot is adducted and plantar flexed

a) Adducted foot
b) Clubfoot
c) Cleft Foot
d) Brachydactyly
e) Congenital foot

ANSWERS

1. C, -Humerus
2. D, -Vertebrae
3. B, -Somtis
4. B, -lateral plate mesoderm
5. C, -Chondroblasts
6. A, -Osteoblasts
7. D, -Chondroblasts
8. E, -Osteoclasts
9. C, -Embryonic skeletal ossification
10. B, -Intramembrannous ossification
11. C, -Fontanelles
12. C, -Osteoblasts & Osteoclasts
13. B, -Neural crest & Paraxial mesoderm
14. B, -Mandible
15. A, -Malleus & incus
16. B, -Ear ossicles
17. B, -Nucles pulposus
18. B, -Periosteum
19. A, -Apical ectoderm ridge
20. C, -Diaphysis
21. D, -Epiphysial plate
22. D, -Diaphysial-epiphysial junction

23. False
24. False
25. True
26. False
27. True
28. False
29. C-Acromegaly

30. B, -Spina bifida
31. C, -Scloliosis
32. A, -Craniosynostosis
33. E, -Sternomelia
34. C, -Spina bifida cystic
35. B, -Clubfoot

Endocrine System

1

Along with the nervous system, the _____ system coordinates the various activities of body parts.
A) digestive
B) endocrine
C) circulatory
D) respiratory
E) excretory

2

A moth sex attractant would be a _____.
A) hormone
B) neurotransmitter
C) pheromone
D) steroid

3

_____ are chemical messengers that are produced in one body region but affect a different body region.
A) Enzymes
B) Endocrines
C) Neurotransmitters
D) Nucleic acids
E) Hormones

4

The endocrine system is quicker than the nervous system.
A) True
B) False

5

Certain cells respond to one hormone and not to another, depending on their receptors.
- A)   True
- B)   False

6

Endocrine glands secrete hormones into the bloodstream for transport to target organs.
- A)   True
- B)   False

7

Hormones are substances that fall into two basic categories:_____.
- A)   stimulator hormones and receptor hormones
- B)   proteins and sugars
- C)   male hormones and female hormones
- D)   non-steroid (peptide) hormones and steroid hormones
- E)   inter-organ and inter-organismic

8

Non-steroid hormones are produced by the adrenal glands, the ovaries, and the testes.
- A)   True
- B)   False

9

The receptors for non-steroid peptide hormones are on the _____.
- A)   plasma membrane
- B)   nuclear envelope
- C)   DNA receptor complex
- D)   peptide chain

10

Non-steroid peptide hormones enter the cell.

A) True
B) False

11

Steroid hormones do NOT bind to plasma membrane receptors.
  A) True
  B) False

12

Steroid hormones lead to the _____ .
  A) destruction of normal DNA
  B) replication of hormones by the cell DNA
  C) synthesis of new enzymes
  D) alteration of the Krebs cycle
  E) better health and longer life

13

The pituitary is located beneath the thalamus in the brain.
  A) True
  B) False

14

The hypothalamus regulates _____ .
  A) heart rate
  B) body temperature
  C) water balance
  D) glandular secretions
  E) all of the above

15

The pituitary gland is divided into two portions: the posterior pituitary and the anterior pituitary.
  A) True
  B) False

16

The posterior pituitary stores and secretes _____.
   A)   ADH and oxytocin
   B)   growth hormone and gonadotropin-releasing hormone
   C)   estrogen and testosterone
   D)   aldosterone and cortisone
   E)   adrenalin and insulin

17

ADH promotes the expulsion of water from the collecting duct, a portion of the nephron.
   A)   True
   B)   False

18

The function(s) of oxytocin is/are to _____.
   A)   cause the uterus to contract
   B)   induce labor
   C)   stimulate the release of milk from the mother's mammary glands when her baby is
nursing.
   D)   all of the above

19

Hypothalamic releasing and release-inhibiting hormones are transported from the hypothalamus
to the anterior pituitary by way of _____.
   A)   the general bloodstream
   B)   a portal system of blood vessels directly connecting the two organs
   C)   direct contact between the two organs
   D)   a cascade of release-inhibit-release-etc. interactions

20

Hormones produced by the anterior pituitary that have a direct effect on the body, rather than
trigger another gland, are _____.
   A)   GH, prolactin, and MSH
   B)   TSH, ACTH, and gonadotropic hormones
   C)   testosterone and estrogen
   D)   FH, LSH and progesterone

21

GH promotes _____.
   A)   cell division
   B)   protein synthesis
   C)   bone growth
   D)   all of the above

22

Which hormone dramatically affects physical appearance?
   A)   gonadotropin-releasing hormone
   B)   growth
   C)   steroid
   D)   male and female

23

If the production of GH increases in an adult after full height has been attained, only certain bones respond and result in acromegaly.
   A)   True
   B)   False

24

Prolactin is produced in quantity throughout every person's life.
   A)   True
   B)   False

25

In humans, MSH (melanocyte-stimulating hormone) _____.
   A)   regulates primary skin color
   B)   causes the thyroid to produce thyroxin
   C)   governs the rate of tanning
   D)   concentration is very low

26

An overproduction of GH in adults causes a condition called _____.
- A)   hyperthyroidism
- B)   acromegaly
- C)   a pituitary giant

27

The parathyroid glands are located _____ .
- A)   below the thyroid, hence the name "para"
- B)   above the thyroid, hence the name "para"
- C)   imbedded in the posterior surface of the thyroid gland
- D)   distant from the thyroid but named because there are two and they resemble the thyroid glands

28

The thyroid gland is attached to the trachea just above the larynx.
- A)   True
- B)   False

29

If _____ is lacking in the diet, the thyroid gland enlarges, producing a goiter.
- A)   thyroxin
- B)   iron
- C)   iodine
- D)   calcium
- E)   phosphorus

30

Thyroxine and triiodothyronine, the thyroid hormones, do not have a specific target organ; instead, they stimulate most of the cells of the body to metabolize at a faster rate.
- A)   True
- B)   False

31

If the thyroid fails to develop properly from childhood, a condition called _____ results.

A) goiter
B) cretinism
C) acromegaly
D) pituitary dwarfism
E) myxedema

32

Hypothyroidism in adults produces a condition called _____ .
    A) goiter
    B) cretinism
    C) acromegaly
    D) pituitary dwarfism
    E) myxedema

33

In addition to thyroxine and triiodothyronine, the thyroid gland produces _____ .
    A) TSH
    B) ACTH
    C) calcitonin
    D) FSH
    E) gonadotropin-releasing hormone

34

Calcitonin _____ .
    A) regulates the calcium level in blood
    B) is balanced by the action of parathyroid hormone
    C) increases the deposit of calcium in bone
    D) all of the above

35

Parathyroid hormone (PTH) _____ .
    A) stops the absorption of calcium from the intestine
    B) stimulates the release of calcium by the kidneys
    C) causes blood calcium level to decrease
    D) causes blood phosphate level to decrease
    E) all of the above

36

If insufficient PTH is produced, the blood calcium level drops, resulting in _____.
- A) reduced growth in childhood or parathyroid dwarfism
- B) tetany, where the body shakes from continuous muscle contraction
- C) osteoporosis
- D) blood clotting
- E) exophthalmic goiter

37

In tetany, the body shakes from continuous muscle contraction.
- A) True
- B) False

38

Calcium plays an important role in _____.
- A) neural conduction
- B) muscle contraction
- C) blood clotting
- D) all of the above

39

The adrenal glands consist of _____.
- A) the inner and outer layer of the kidney
- B) the inner medulla and the outer cortex
- C) lower adrenal and upper paradrenal sections
- D) ACTH and BCTH sections

40

The medulla and the cortex portions of the adrenal glands function together as a physiological unit.
- A) True
- B) False

41

The adrenal medulla secretes _____ under conditions of stress.
>A) norepinephrine
>B) epinephrine
>C) both of the above

42

The adrenal _____ secretes a small amount of both sex hormones.
>A) medulla
>B) cortex
>C) accessory gland

43

Cortisol is a _____.
>A) sex hormone
>B) glucocorticoid
>C) mineralocorticoid

44

ACTH controls the secretion of _____.
>A) cortisol
>B) aldosterone
>C) epinephrine
>D) testosterone

45

Aldosterone regulates the blood sodium and potassium levels.
>A) True
>B) False

46

The primary target organ of aldosterone is _____.
>A) the liver
>B) the pancreas
>C) the kidney

D)   all of the above

47

The heart produces a hormone that acts to increase aldosterone.
   A)   True
   B)   False

48

Low levels of adrenal cortex hormones result in _____.
   A)   Addison disease
   B)   Cushing syndrome
   C)   diabetes
   D)   tetany
   E)   goiter

49

A person with Addison disease _____.
   A)   is unable to replenish blood glucose levels under stressful conditions
   B)   develops dramatically more male features
   C)   develops a rounded face and edema
   D)   has overgrowth of hands and face
   E)   all of the above

50

A person with Cushing syndrome has a tendency toward diabetes mellitus.
   A)   True
   B)   False

51

The pancreas has both exocrine and endocrine tissue.
   A)   True
   B)   False

52

The pancreatic endocrine tissues are called pancreatic islets.
- A) True
- B) False

53

There is/are _____ type(s) of diabetes mellitus.
- A) one
- B) three
- C) two
- D) five

54

The pancreatic islets produce _____.
- A) insulin and glucagon
- B) pancreatin
- C) ACTH and aldosterone
- D) pancreatic digestive enzymes

55

Insulin functions to _____.
- A) promote the storage of nutrients
- B) lower the blood glucose level by stimulating liver, fat and muscle cells to metabolize glucose
- C) stimulate uptake of glucose by cells
- D) all of the above

56

Glucagon increases the action of insulin.
- A) True
- B) False

57

In _____ diabetes the pancreas is NOT producing insulin.
- A) type I

B) type II
C) type III
D) all forms of

58

It is believed that type I diabetes is brought on by an environmental agent, probably a virus.
A) True
B) False

59

Type II diabetes usually occurs in people who are obese and inactive.
A) True
B) False

60

In type II diabetes, insulin is produced but the live and muscle cells do NOT respond to it.
A) True
B) False

61

The _____ are the male sex hormones.
A) androgens
B) estrogens
C) aldosterones
D) insulins
E) pheromones

62

Anabolic steroids are _____ forms of testosterone.
A) natural
B) synthetic
C) super-active
D) ineffective

63

The thymus increases in size with aging.
    A)   True
    B)   False

64

The thymus aids the differentiation of _____ cells.
    A)   red blood
    B)   B
    C)   T
    D)   cancerous

65

The _____ produces the hormone melatonin.
    A)   pituitary gland
    B)   pineal gland
    C)   thyroid gland
    D)   pancreatic gland
    E)   hypothalamus

66

Melatonin is involved with circadian rhythms.
    A)   True
    B)   False

67

The family of chemical messengers that causes the pain and discomfort of menstruation are

_____.
    A)   ADH
    B)   Progesterones
    C)   Prostaglandins
    D)   Steroids

68

_____ helps reduce pain because it inhibits the synthesis of prostaglandins.
A) Cyanide
B) Acetaminophen
C) Serotonin
D) Aspirin

ANSWERS

1. B	24. B	47. B
2. C	25. D	48. A
3. E	26. B	49. A
4. B	27. C	50. A
5. A	28. B	51. A
6. A	29. C	52. A
7. D	30. A	53. C
8. B	31. B	54. A
9. A	32. E	55. C
10. B	33. C	56. B
11. A	34. D	57. A
12. B	35. D	58. A
13. A	36. B	59. A
14. E	37. A	60. A
15. A	38. D	61. A
16. A	39. B	62. B
17. B	40. B	63. B
18. D	41. C	64. C
19. B	42. B	65. B
20. A	43. B	66. A
21. D	44. A	67. C
22. B	45. A	68. D
23. A	46. C	

Circulatory system

Please answer all questions

1

The liquid part of blood after the fibrinogen is removed is
- A) plasma
- B) lymph
- C) serum
- D) puss

2

Unlike any other vertebrates, the erythrocytes of mammals
- A) undergo erythropoiesis
- B) are capable of phagocytosis
- C) secrete antibodies
- D) are multinucleate

3

The tissue layer common to all blood vessels is the
- A) circular smooth muscle
- B) endothelium
- C) longitudinal striated muscle
- D) connective tissue

4

Atria contract
- A) just before diastole
- B) during diastole
- C) right after the systole
- D) during the systole

5

The heartbeat begins with the depolarization of the
A)   atrioventricular node
B)   bundle of His
C)   sinoatrial node
D)   Purkinje fibers

6

Which of the following contains oxygenated blood in an adult human?
A)   right atrium
B)   pulmonary artery
C)   pulmonary vein
D)   all of the above
E)   none of the above

7

The sinoatrial node is derived from the more primitive
A)   ventricle
B)   bundle of His
C)   conus arteriosus
D)   tricuspid valve
E)   sinus venosus

8

Water that diffuses out of the blood plasma is returned to the cardiovascular system by the
A)   hepatic vein
B)   aorta
C)   lymphatic system
D)   megakaryocytes
E)   septum

9

Which of the following is the most muscular chamber in a bird's heart or a mammal's heart?
A)   the right atrium
B)   the left atrium
C)   the left ventricle

D) the right ventricle
E) all are equally muscular

10

In which type of heart is there mixing of oxygenated and deoxygenated blood?
A) fish
B) frog
C) crocodile
D) all of the above
E) none of the above

11

Which of the following statements about circulatory systems is true?
A) Hormones are transported in the blood.
B) All invertebrates have an open circulatory system.
C) Capillaries have thicker walls than veins do.
D) The systemic circulation carries blood to and from the lungs.
E) All of the above are true.

12

Materials are exchanged between the blood and the surrounding tissues in the
A) arteries
B) veins
C) capillaries
D) all of the above
E) none of the above

13

Oxygenated blood leaves the human heart via the
A) pulmonary vein
B) pulmonary artery
C) vena cava
D) aorta
E) respiratory circuit

14

The innermost tissue layer of arteries is composed of
- A) smooth muscle
- B) Purkinje fibers
- C) connective tissue
- D) elastic fibers
- E) endothelium

15

The lymphatic system
- A) is an open circulatory system
- B) contains one-way valves
- C) returns fluids to the bloodstream
- D) all of the above
- E) none of the above

16

Which of the following is a type of leukocyte?
- A) macrophage
- B) eosinophil
- C) monocyte
- D) all of the above
- E) none of the above

17

Which is the most common type of blood cell in a healthy human?
- A) erythrocytes
- B) monocytes
- C) lymphocytes
- D) eosinophils
- E) basophils

18

Which of the following is a function of the vertebrate circulatory system?
- A) temperature regulation
- B) transport metabolic wastes
- C) provide immune defense

D) transport oxygen and carbon dioxide
E) all of the above

19

During heavy exercise, which of the following should happen?
A) decreased stroke volume
B) decreased heart rate
C) vasodilation of blood vessels in skin
D) all of the above
E) none of the above

20

Interstitial fluid is derived from fluid that is forced out of the
A) venule end of capillaries
B) arteriole end of capillaries
C) lymph vessels
D) arteries
E) veins

21

Which one of the following is not part of the cardiovascular system?
A) arteries
B) heart
C) blood
D) veins
E) All of the above are part of the cardiovascular system.

22

Compared to arteries, arterioles:
A) are smaller in diameter
B) can be relaxed by hormones
C) collapse when empty
D) a and b are correct.
E) All of the above statements are correct.

23

The transfer of oxygen to the body's cells takes place in the:
A)   arteries
B)   arterioles
C)   capillaries
D)   venules
E)   a, b, and c are correct.

24

Unidirectional valves that prevent the blood from flowing backward are found in the:
A)   arteries
B)   veins
C)   capillaries
D)   all of the above
E)   none of the above

25

Fluid is driven through the lymphatic system by:
A)   contraction of the walls of the lymphatic vessels
B)   pressure created by the pumping of the heart
C)   contractions of the lymph nodes
D)   squeezing of the lymphatic vessels by the body's muscles
E)   a combination of all of the above

26

The lymphatic system is important because it:
A)   collects liquid lost from the circulatory system
B)   returns proteins to circulation
C)   transports fats
D)   carries bacteria to the lymph nodes for destruction
E)   does all of the above

27

Plasma is made up of water and _____.
A)   metabolites and wastes
B)   salts and ions
C)   proteins

D)   all of the above
E)   none of the above

28

The component of blood that is responsible for clotting is:
   A)   platelets
   B)   erythrocytes
   C)   neutrophils
   D)   basophils
   E)   none of the above

29

Which one of the following series represents the correct path of blood circulation?
   A)   left atrium, left ventricle, lungs, right atrium, right ventricle, body
   B)   right atrium, right ventricle, lungs, left atrium, left ventricle, body
   C)   left atrium, left ventricle, right atrium, right ventricle, lungs, body
   D)   right atrium, lungs, right ventricle, left atrium, body, left ventricle
   E)   left atrium, lungs, left ventricle, body, right atrium, right ventricle

30

The rhythmic beating of the heart is initiated by the:
   A)   Purkinje fibers
   B)   bundle of His
   C)   atrioventricular node
   D)   sinoatrial node
   E)   right ventricle

31

The "lub" of the "lub-dub" sound the heart makes is caused by the:
   A)   closing of the mitral and tricuspid valves
   B)   closing of the pulmonary and aortic valves
   C)   sound of blood rushing into the atria
   D)   sound of blood rushing into the ventricles
   E)   none of the above

32

Hemoglobin, contained in leukocytes, transports oxygen throughout the body.
- A) True
- B) False

33

Pulmonary veins carry blood that is rich in oxygen.
- A) True
- B) False

34

The brain regulates the rate at which you breathe by monitoring the amount of oxygen in the blood.
- A) True
- B) False

35

Blood serum contains red but not white blood cells.
- A) True
- B) False

ANSWERS

1. C	13. D	25. D
2. A	14. E	26. E
3. B	15. D	27. D
4. B	16. D	28. A
5. C	17. A	29. B
6. C	18. E	30. D
7. E	19. C	31. B
8. C	20. B	32. B
9. C	21. C	33. A
10. B	22. D	34. B
11. A	23. C	35. B
12. C	24. B	

1.   What is another name for a T lymphocytes?

     A.   T-cells.
     B.   B-cells.
     C.   Hemoglobin.
     D.   Red blood cell.

2.   What is the circulatory system?

     A.   The system that helps your body breathe.
     B.   Your body's muscles. (Your Answer)
     C.   Your body's nerves.
     D.   Your body's blood transporting system. (Correct Answer)

3.   What is the smallest blood vessel?

     A.   Arteries.
     B.   Capillaries.
     C.   Veins.

4.   The heart has how many chambers?

     A.   1
     B.   2
     C.   3
     D.   4
     E.   5

5.   The left and right sides of your heart work ___.

     A.   Together.
     B.   Seperately.
     C.   Against each other.
     D.   None of the above.

6.   With circulation, the heart provides your body with:

A. Oxygen
B. Nutrients
C. A way to get rid of waste
D. All of the above.

7. The heart is located near the center of your....

A. Stomach.
B. Head.
C. Chest.
D. Back.

8. What do we call platelet plugs?

A. Scabs.
B. Band aids.
C. Cuts.
D. Bruises.

9. Red blood cells transport _____.

A. Oxygen.
B. Carbon dioxide.
C. Nitrogen.
D. Hydrogen.

10. When in the lungs, the _____ leaves the blood

A. Oxygen
B. Carbon Dioxide
C. Nitrogen.
D. Phosphorus.

11. What links the arteries to the veins?

A. Muscle.
B. Capillaries.
C. Aorta.

12.   The right side of the heart pumps the blood ____ the heart ____ the lungs.

    A.   To, from
    B.   From, to
    C.   To, to
    D.   From, from

13.   What is your heart made of?

    A.   Skin.
    B.   Tissue.
    C.   Muscle.

14.   Where do arteries carry blood?

    A.   To the heart.
    B.   Away from the heart.

15.   Plasma is about ____ percent water.

    A.   60
    B.   70
    C.   80
    D.   90
    E.   95

16.   Which of the following is NOT a function of white blood cells?

    A.   Guard against infection.
    B.   Fight parasites.
    C.   Attack bacteria.
    D.   Carry oxygen.

17.   Which of the following could be compared to soliders?

    A.   Your heart.
    B.   Red blood cells.
    C.   White blood cells.
    D.   Your lungs.

18.   Where to the veins carry blood?

    A.   To the heart.
    B.   Away from the heart.

19.   What divides the left side of the heart from the left side?

    A.   Septum.
    B.   Atrium.
    C.   Ventricles.
    D.   Wall.

20.   The movement of blood through the heart and body is called circulation.

True or False.

    A.   True.
    B.   False

21.   What color are white blood cells?

    A.   White.
    B.   Red.
    C.   Yellow.
    D.   Colorless.

22.   What is your strongest muscle?

    A.   Your lungs.
    B.   Your legs.
    C.   Your arms.
    D.   Your heart.

23.   What is blood clotting made possible by?

    A.   Platelets.
    B.   Hemoglobin.
    C.   Lymphocytes.

D.   Plasma.

24.   What is the largest blood vessel?

   A.   Aorta.
   B.   Artery.
   C.   Capillary.
   D.   Veins.

25.   What happens when blood pools in the veins?

   A.   You fall over.
   B.   You become paralyzed.
   C.   You get varicose veins.

26.   What is the most common type of blood cells?

   A.   White blood cells.
   B.   Platelets.
   C.   Red blood cells.

27.   White blood cells contain a _____, while red blood cells do not.

   A.   Nucleus.
   B.   Brain.
   C.   Red color.
   D.   Hemoglobin.

28.   The heart is about the size of your...

   A.   Leg.
   B.   Brain.
   C.   Arm.
   D.   Fist.

29.
The circulatory system is composed of...

   A.   The heart, blood, and blood vessels.

B. The heart, the brain, and the lungs.
C. The lungs, the blood, and the blood vessels.
D. The brain, the heart, and the blood vessels.

30.
Where is plasma found?

A. In blood.
B. In urine.
C. In your brain.
D. In your muscles.

ANSWERS

1. A	16. D
2. D	17. C
3. B	18. A
4. D	19. A
5. A	20. A
6. D	21. D
7. C	22. D
8. A	23. A
9. A	24. A
10. B	25. C
11. B	26. C
12. B	27. A
13. C	28. D
14. B	29. A
15. D	30. A

Quiz 3.

1)   The outermost layer of the pericardium, which consists of inelastic dense irregular connective tissue, is called the

     A.   Pericardial cavity
     B.   Parietal layer of pericardium
     C.   Fibrous pericardium
     D.   Epicardium
     E.   Serous pericardium

2)   This consists of mesothelium and connective tissue.

     A.   Fibrous pericardium
     B.   Endocardium
     C.   Pericardial cavity
     D.   Epicardium
     E.   Myocardium

3)   Which layer consists of cardiac muscle tissue?

     A.   Epicardium
     B.   Pericardium
     C.   Hypocardium
     D.   Myocardium
     E.   Endocardium

4)   This pouch-like structure increases the total filling capacity of the atrium.

     A.   Ventricle
     B.   Coronary sulcus
     C.   Fossa ovalis
     D.   Interatrial septum
     E.   Auricle

5)   These muscular ridges are found on the anterior wall of the right atrium and extend into the auricles.

     A.   Papillary muscles
     B.   Trabeculae carneae

C. Chordae tendinae
D. Coronary sulci
E. Pectinate muscles

6) What types of tissue comprise the valves of the heart?

A. Dense connective tissue
B. Areolar connective tissue
C. Hyaline cartilage
D. Cardiac muscle tissue

7) From the left ventricle, where does blood pass?

A. Aortic semilunar valve
B. Pulmonary trunk
C. Right ventricle
D. Right atrium
E. Bicuspid valve

8) In a fetus, this structure temporarily shunts blood from the pulmonary trunk into the aorta.

A. Foramen ovale
B. Trabeculae carnae
C. Fossa ovalis
D. Descending aorta
E. Ductus arteriosus

9) As each ventricle contracts where does blood move?

A. Into the apex
B. Through the apex
C. Into an artery
D. Through an atrioventricular valve
E. Into a vein

10) As each atrium contracts where does blood move?

A. Into a vein
B. Into an artery

C. Through an atrioventricular valve
D. Through a semilunar valve
E. Into an auricle

11) Which valve below prevents blood from flowing back into the right ventricle?

A. Pulmonary valve
B. Tricuspid valve
C. Aortic valve
D. Pulmonary vein
E. Bicuspid valve

12) In this disorder the aortic valve is narrowed.

A. Mitral valve prolapse
B. Mitral insufficiency
C. Aortic insufficiency
D. Aortic stenosis
E. Rheumatic fever

13) This heart structure(s) carries deoxygenated blood.

A. Left atrium and ventricle
B. Left atrium only
C. Right ventricle only
D. Right atrium and ventricle
E. Left atrium and right ventricle

14) Cardiac muscle fibers electrically connect to neighboring fibers by

A. Intermediate discs
B. Gap junctions
C. Contractile fibers
D. Chordae tendinae
E. Desmosomes

15) This is a the correct sequence of structures that allows the normal sequence of excitation to progress through the heart.

A. Bundle of His, SA node, AV node, Purkinje fibers

B.   Sinoatrial (SA), Purkinje fibers, AV node, Bundle of His
C.   Purkinje fibers, AV node, SA node, Bundle of His
D.   SA node, AV node, Bundle of His, Purkinje fibers
E.   Bundle of His, Purkinje fibers, Atrioventricular (AV) node

16)   This term refers to the period of time during a cardiac cycle when contraction occurs and blood pressure rises.

A.   Systole
B.   Repolarization
C.   Fibrillation
D.   Filling
E.   Diastole

17)   During which of following periods does the largest volume of blood enter the arteries?

A.   Atrial diastole
B.   Ventricular diastole
C.   Atrial systole
D.   Ventricular systole

18)   The second heart sound (dupp) closely follows which of the events listed below.

A.   Semilunar valves opening
B.   Atrioventricular valves opening
C.   Atrioventricular valves closing
D.   Semilunar valves closing
E.   Valvular stenosis

19)   This part of the heart can initiate a contraction and can set a constant heart rate of about 100 beats per minute.

A.   Cardiovascular center
B.   Sinoatrial SA node
C.   Cardiac accelerator nerves
D.   Chemoreceptors
E.   Proprioceptors

20)   Which of the below reduces heart rate.

A. Increased sympathetic stimulation
B. Increased Norepinephrine hormone
C. Increased Thyroid hormone
D. Increased calcium levels
E. Increased potassium levels

21) This part of the brain contains the cardiovascular center that regulates heart rate.

A. Medulla oblongata
B. Thalamus
C. Cerebellum
D. Midbrain
E. Cerebrum

22) Which of the below factors would increase Stroke volume?

A. Increased preload, increased afterload, decreased contractility
B. Increased preload, increased afterload, increased contractility
C. Decreased preload, decreased afterload, decreased contractility
D. Decreased preload, increased afterload, increased contractility
E. Increased preload, decreased afterload, increased contractility

USE THIS IMAGE TO ANSWER QUESTIONS 23, 24 AND 25

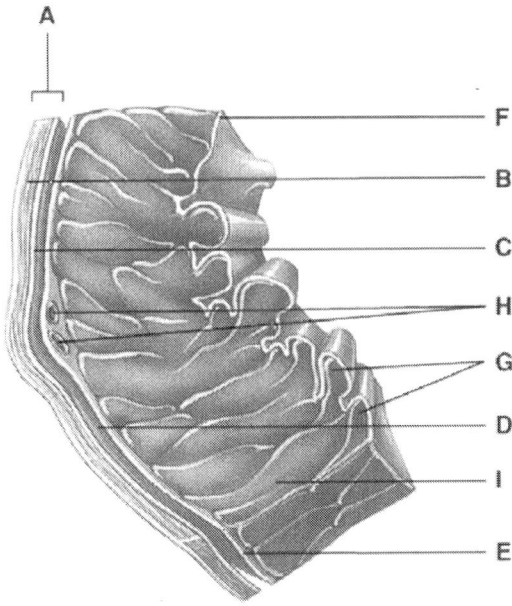

23) This portion of the heart wall is responsible for the pumping action.

A. E
B. I
C. F
D. G
E. H

24) This is comprised of a thin layer of endothelium overlying a thin layer of connective tissue.

A. E
B. C
C. D
D. G
E. F

25) Which layer of the pericardium consists of dense irregular connective tissue?

A. E
B. A
C. B
D. C
E. D

USE THE FOLLOWING DIAGRAM TO ANSWER QUESTIONS 26, 27 AND 28

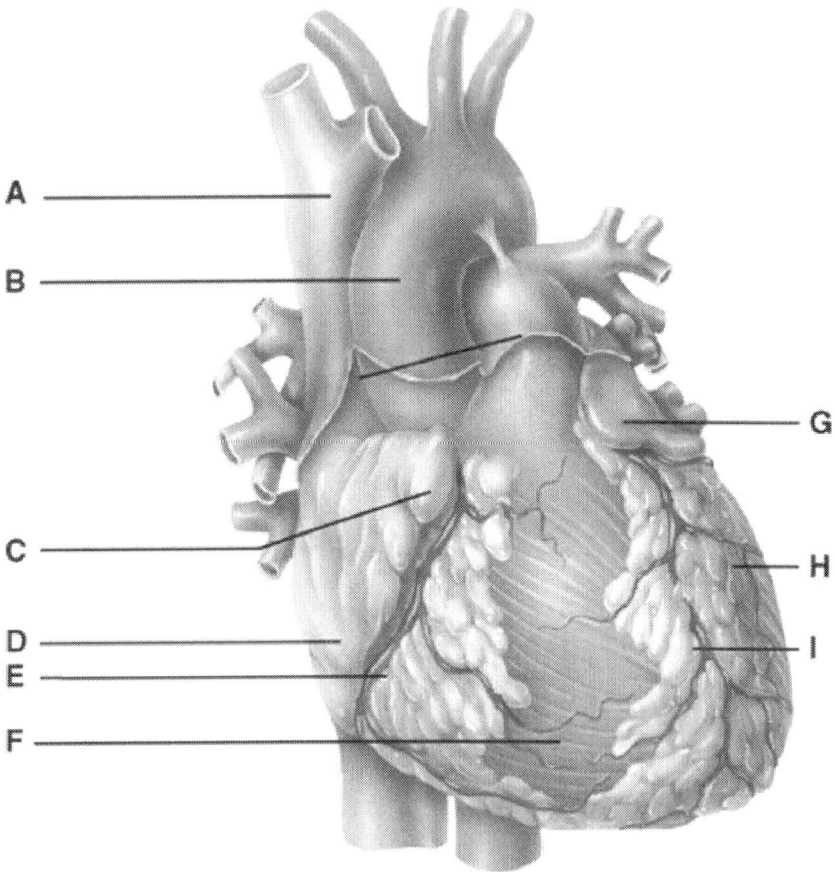

26) In the diagram, where is the coronary sulcus?

A. I
B. H
C. G

D.   E
E.   G

27)   In the diagram, where is the left auricle of left atrium?

A.   H
B.   I
C.   C
D.   F
E.   G

28)   In the diagram, these contain coronary blood vessels and a variable amount of fat.

A.   F and H
B.   A and B
C.   C and G
D.   E and I
E.   D and F

USE THE FOLLOWING IMAGE TO ANSWER QUESTIONS 29 AND 30

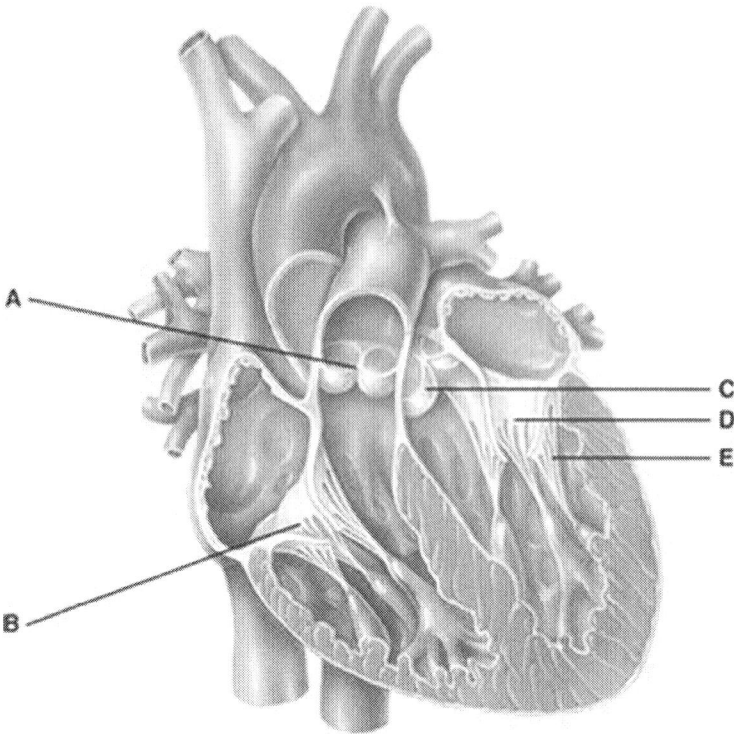

29) Which of the structures in the diagram below represent semilunar valves?

    A.   B
    B.   D
    C.   E
    D.   A & C
    E.   NONE OF THE ABOVE

30) In the diagram, where is the atrioventricular valve?

    A.   B
    B.   D
    C.   A
    D.   B & D
    E.   B,D, and A

31) The structure indicated is the

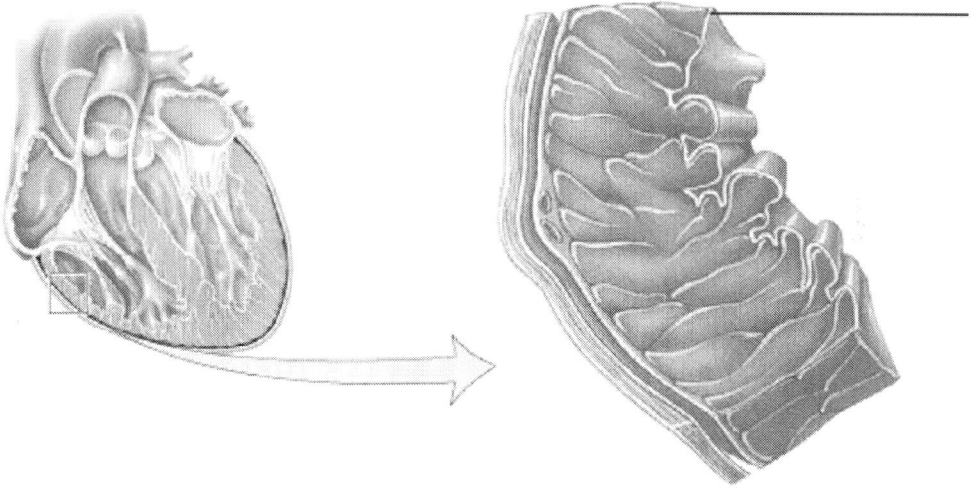

A.   Epicardium.
B.   Fibrous pericardium.
C.   Myocardium.
D.   Endocardium.
E.   Parietal layer of the serous pericardium.

32) The purpose of the structure indicated is to

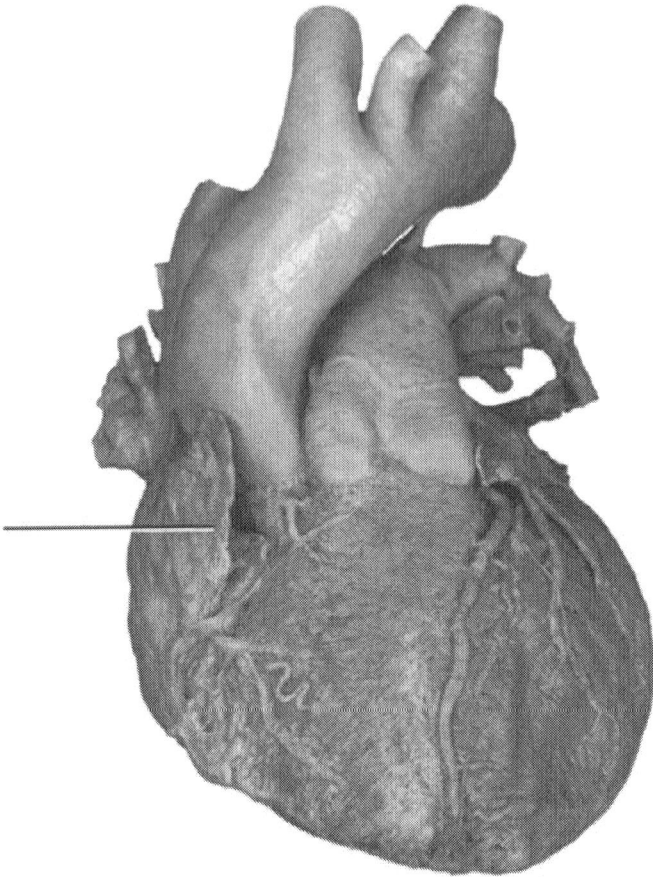

A.   Protect the heart from stress.
B.   Slightly increase the capacity of the atrium. (Your Answer)
C.   Serve as an entry point for the superior vena cava.
D.   A and B.
E.   A, B, and C.

33)   Which of the following statements is NOT correct?

A.   The walls of the ventricles are thicker because the ventricles pump blood under higher pressure over greater distances.
B.   The walls of the atria are thicker because the atria receive blood under pressure.

C.   The wall of the right ventricle is thinner than that of the left ventricle because the right side of the heart pumps blood a shorter distance at lower pressure.

D.   Although the right side of the heart has a smaller workload, the right and left ventricle simultaneously eject the same amount of blood.

E.   All of the above are correct.

34)   The function of the fibrous skeleton of the heart is to

A.   Provide a structural foundation for the heart valves.
B.   Act as an insertion point for bundles of cardiac muscle fibers.
C.   Serve as an electrical insulator between the atria and ventricles.
D.   A and B are correct.
E.   A, B, and C are correct.

35)   Prolapse of the atrioventricular valves is prevented by

A.   Contraction of the pectinate muscles.
B.   Contraction of the papillary muscles.
C.   Contraction of the chordae tendineae.
D.   The fibrous skeleton of the heart.
E.   Increasing blood pressure in the ventricles.

36)   The semilunar valves open when pressure in the right and left ventricles exceeds that in the pulmonary trunk and aorta, respectively.

A.   True
B.   False

37)   Collateral circulation in the heart

A.   May allow bypass of a blocked coronary artery.
B.   Branches directly from the ascending aorta.
C.   Directly returns blood to the inferior vena cava.
D.   Allows bypass of the pulmonary circulation before birth.
E.   Helps return blood from the lungs to the left atrium.

38)   Reperfusion of cardiac muscle after blockage of a coronary artery may cause as much or more damage to the myocardium than did the lack of oxygen.

A.   True
B.   False

39) The intercalated discs seen in cardiac myocytes

    A.   Have desmosomes which help to hold the muscle fibers together.
    B.   Have gap junctions which allow action potentials to conduct from one muscle
fiber to the next.
    C.   Are the result of actin/myosin overlap.
    D.   A and B are correct.
    E.   A, B, and C are correct.

40) If the SA node is damaged, the AV node will take over and the parasympathetic division of the autonomic nervous system will help to maintain a normal heart rate between 60-80 beats per minute.

    A.   True
    B.   False

41) An electrocardiogram can help determine all of the following except:

    A.   If the conduction pathway is functioning normally
    B.   All the above can be determined during an ECG
    C.   A cause of chest pain
    D.   If a heart attack has occurred
    E.   if the heart has enlarged

42) Which wave is matched correctly with the heart's activity?

    A.   QRS complex – atrial repolarization
    B.   P wave – ventricular repolarization
    C.   T wave – ventricular depolarization
    D.   S-T segment – the ventricles are depolarized

43) What is occurring during isovolumetric contraction?

    A.   Both atria are ejecting blood at the same time
    B.   The amount of blood in each atria is the same
    C.   The semilunar valves are open and the AV valves are closed
    D.   The point at which all blood has been ejected from the ventricles
    E.   All four valves are closed

44) More blood flows through the coronary arteries during ventricular diastole than ventricular systole.

A.　True
B.　False

45)　Which phases of a heartbeat shown in the figure below involve repolarization of the atria and the ventricles?

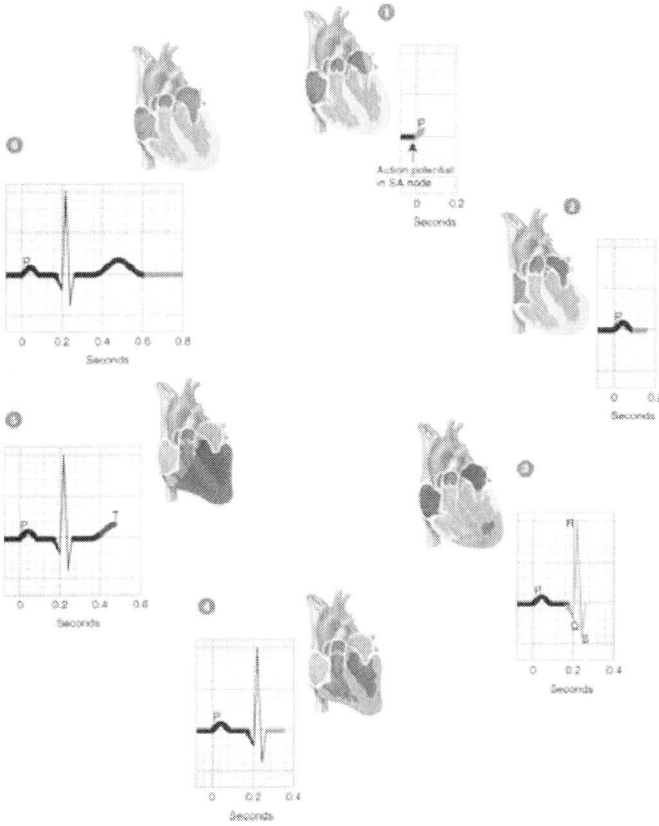

A.　1, 2, 3, and 4
B.　2 and 4
C.　1 and 3
D.　2, 4 and 6
E.　4 and 6

USE THE IMAGE TO ANSWER QUESTIONS 46 AND 47

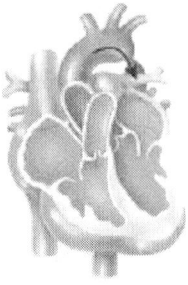

A

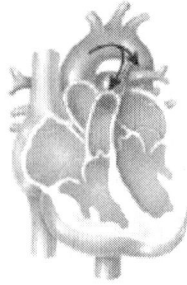

B

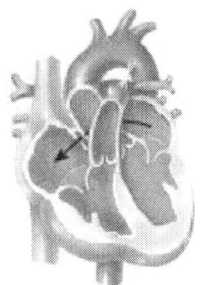

C

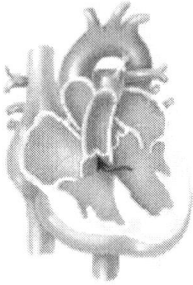

D

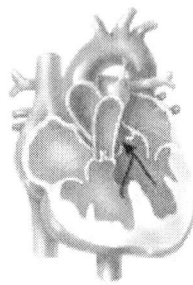

E

46) Which of the following represents coarctation of the aorta?

A. A
B. B
C. E
D. C
E. D

Incorrect

47) Which of the following represents an atrial septal defect?

A. A
B. C
C. B
D. D
E. E

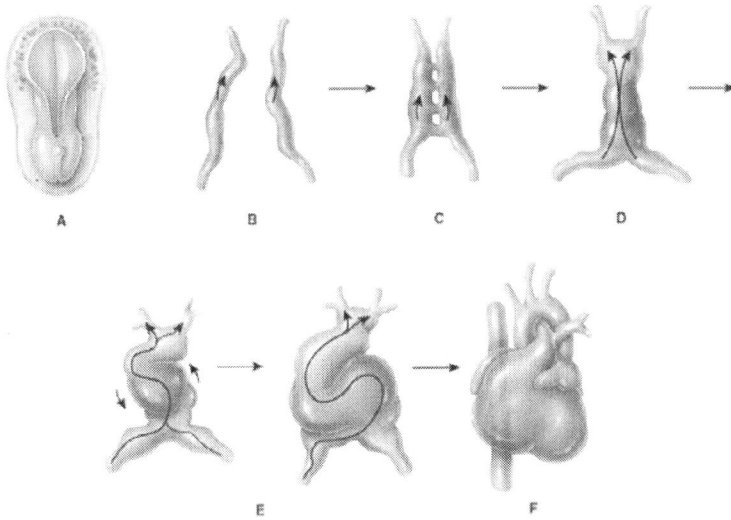

48) Which of the following represents the formation of the primitive heart tube?

A. D
B. E
C. B
D. A
E. C

49) Which of the following represents formation of the endocardial tubes?

A. B
B. C
C. E
D. A
E. D

50) Isovolumetric contraction and isovolumetric relaxation both occur when all four valves are closed.

A. True

B.   False

51)   Which statement is not true regarding heart sounds?

A.   S4 occurs during atrial filling and is not usually heard
B.   S3 occurs during ventricular filling
C.   S1 is caused by closing of the AV valves
D.   The second sound is due to the SL valves closing
E.   S2 is louder and a little longer than the first sound

52)   The amount of blood ejected from either ventricle every minute is called:

A.   Stroke volume
B.   Heart rate
C.   End-diastolic volume
D.   Cardiac output
E.   Afterload

53)   The stroke volume at rest is what percentage of end-diastolic volume?

A.   100%
B.   80-90%
C.   50-60%
D.   40-50%
E.   0%

54)   The Frank-Starling law of the heart states:

A.   The greater the afterload the lower the pressure that must be overcome
B.   The greater the stroke volume the greater the heart rate
C.   The more the heart is stretched pre-contraction the stronger the force of contraction
D.   The lower the preload on the heart the greater the force of contraction
E.   The faster the heart rate the greater the volume of blood pumped

55)   The cardiac reserve would be lower in a well-trained athlete than a sedentary individual.

A.   True
B.   False

56)   Which of the following statements is false in reference to heart regulation?

A.   At rest, parasympathetic stimulation predominates
B.   Sympathetic stimulation triggers the release of norepinephrine
C.   The movement of limbs is monitored by proprioceptors
D.   Baroreceptors measure the amount of sodium ions present in the blood
E.   Parasympathetic fibers travel via the vagus nerve

57)   Resting cardiac output (CO) in a well-conditioned athlete is about the same as in a healthy untrained person.

A.   True
B.   False

ANSWERS

1. C	21. A	41. B
2. D	22. E	42. D
3. D	23. B	43. E
4. E	24. E	44. A
5. E	25. B	45. A
6. A	26. D	46. A
7. A	27. E	47. B
8. E	28. D	48. E
9. C	29. D	49. B
10. C	30. D	50. A
11. A	31. D	51. E
12. D	32. B	52. D
13. D	33. B	53. C
14. B	34. E	54. C
15. D	35. B	55. B
16. A	36. A	56. D
17. D	37. A	57. A
18. D	38. A	
19. B	39. D	
20. E	40. B	

FINAL

QUIZ 1

1

Anatomy is a term, which means the study of _____.
A) physiology
B) morphology
C) cell functions
D) human functions

2

The study dealing with the explanations of how an organ works would be an example of

_____.
A) anatomy
B) cytology
C) telcology
D) physiology

3

The process of turning molecules that are ingested into forms that are compatible with the organism is _____.
A) digestion
B) absorption
C) assimilation
D) circulation

4

The exchanging of gases for the purpose of producing energy is called _____.
A) breathing
B) respiration
C) circulation
D) responsiveness

5

The removal of a compound that the body no longer requires is called ____.
    A)   secretion
    B)   excretion
    C)   movement
    D)   digestion

6

When a nurse takes someone's temperature, they are directly assessing a ____.
    A)   metabolic activity
    B)   sign of illness
    C)   vital sign
    D)   core temperature

7

The following are essential needs of the body except which one?
    A)   water
    B)   chemicals
    C)   set point
    D)   pressure

8

The force that water exerts on a system is referred to as the ____.
    A)   hydrophilic factor
    B)   hydrostatic pressure
    C)   atmospheric pressure
    D)   osmotic pressure

9

The transportation of heat in the body is mainly a property of the ____ it contains.
    A)   food
    B)   oxygen
    C)   water
    D)   pressure

10

The process in which cells and organisms are able to maintain a stable balance of internal and external substances and forces is called _____.

A)   equilibrium
B)   adaptation
C)   adjustment
D)   homeostasis

11

The following is an example of a homeostatic event.

A)   sweating during a test
B)   shivering when it is cold
C)   developing a headache
D)   muscle strain

12

The following are examples of homeostatic parameters or body values except which one?

A)   heart rate
B)   blood pressure
C)   blood glucose levels
D)   insulin production

13

A decrease in blood glucose that causes the inhibition of insulin is an example of _____.

A)   positive feedback
B)   negative feedback
C)   abnormal function
D)   the action of glucagon

14

The following is an example of positive feedback:

A)   glucagon raises blood sugar
B)   insulin lowers blood glucose
C)   a temperature of 100.2F causes a further increase
D)   100.1F is followed by 98.6F

15

A system is defined as a group of _____ that function together.

     A)   cells
     B)   tissues
     C)   molecules
     D)   organs

16

The structures called _____ are intracellular areas with specific living functions.

     A)   inclusions
     B)   organs
     C)   organelles
     D)   macromolecules

17

Proteins and carbohydrates are classified as _____.

     A)   macromolecules
     B)   microbes
     C)   organelles
     D)   atoms

18

The following belong together except which one?

     A)   head
     B)   arm
     C)   neck
     D)   trunk

19

Simple squamous epithelium is a _____ term.

     A)   tissue
     B)   cell
     C)   organ
     D)   pathology

20

The ____ separates the thoracic from abdominal cavities.

    A)   pelvis
    B)   rib cage
    C)   diaphragm
    D)   peritoneum

21

The following belong together except which one?

    A)   brain
    B)   vertebral canal
    C)   spinal cord
    D)   stomach

22

The heart lies specifically in the ____ space.

    A)   thoracic cavity
    B)   mediastinum
    C)   abdominal cavity
    D)   pleural cavity

23

The orbital cavity would contain the ____.

    A)   eyes
    B)   nasal septum
    C)   brain
    D)   teeth

24

The following are correct cavity terms except which one?

    A)   oral
    B)   nasal
    C)   frontal
    D)   middle ear

25

Another name for the cavity in the front or belly side is _____ .
- A)   dorsal
- B)   ventral
- C)   abdominopelvic
- D)   vertebral

26

The _____ membranes surround the lungs.
- A)   pericardial
- B)   mediastinal
- C)   pleural
- D)   peritoneal

27

Which of the following would not be lined by peritoneum?
- A)   heart
- B)   stomach
- C)   intestines
- D)   liver

28

The following are sinus areas except which one?
- A)   frontal
- B)   maxillary
- C)   ethmoid
- D)   cranial

29

The _____ system plays a role in moving fluids, wastes, and bones?
- A)   skeletal
- B)   integumentary
- C)   muscular
- D)   nervous

30

The skin belongs to the _____ system.
- A)　　nervous
- B)　　integumentary
- C)　　circulatory
- D)　　muscular

31

Integration and coordination are properties of the _____ system of organs.
- A)　　nervous
- B)　　circulatory
- C)　　excretory
- D)　　muscular

32

Hormones are chemicals of the _____ system that affect target areas.
- A)　　cardiovascular
- B)　　endocrine
- C)　　exocrine
- D)　　nervous

33

The following belong together except which one?
- A)　　pituitary
- B)　　thyroid
- C)　　brain
- D)　　adrenal

34

The following belong together except which one?
- A)　　trachea
- B)　　bronchi
- C)　　esophagus
- D)　　larynx

35

Parts of the pharynx belong to the _____ and digestive systems.
- A) respiratory
- B) circulatory
- C) nervous
- D) skeletal

36

The larynx is a term in the _____ system.
- A) integumentary
- B) respiratory
- C) digestive
- D) nervous

37

The _____ system returns tissue fluids to the heart.
- A) circulatory
- B) lymphatic
- C) integumentary
- D) histologic

38

The function of the _____ is to remove soluble wastes from the body.
- A) lungs
- B) gastrointestinal tract
- C) kidneys
- D) skin

39

The following are components of the excretory system except which one?
- A) lungs
- B) large intestine
- C) integument
- D) salivary glands

40

The bulbourethral glands would be found in the ____ system.
- A) reproductive
- B) excretory
- C) circulatory
- D) endocrine

41

A tumor on top of the head would be on the ____ surface.
- A) inferior
- B) superior
- C) medial
- D) lateral

42

The navel is located on the ____ surface.
- A) cranial
- B) ventral
- C) dorsal
- D) inferior

43

The wrist is ____ to the fingers with respect to the elbow.
- A) distal
- B) inferior
- C) superior
- D) proximal

44

The wrist is the ____ part of the hand region.
- A) proximal
- B) distal
- C) superior
- D) inferior

45

A medial tumor on the head could be on the ____.
A) ear
B) cheeks
C) nose
D) eye

46

The arms lie on the ____ surface of the trunk.
A) medial
B) lateral
C) distal
D) posterior

47

A ____ section divides the body into right and left.
A) coronal
B) transverse
C) sagittal
D) frontal

48

A ____ section divides an organ into top and bottom.
A) sagittal
B) oblique
C) coronal
D) transverse

49

Which of the following is the same as inguinal?
A) epigastric
B) hypochondriac
C) lumbar
D) iliac

50

The lower ribs are below the ____ region.
        A)   lumbar
        B)   epigastric
        C)   hypogastric
        D)   hypochondriac

51

The central abdominal area is the ____ region.
        A)   iliac
        B)   hypogastric
        C)   peritoneal
        D)   umbilical

52

A ____ fracture occurred in the elbow area.
        A)   dorsum
        B)   buccal
        C)   carpal
        D)   cubital

53

The forearm is a/an ____ area.
        A)   antecubital
        B)   antebrachial
        C)   cephalic
        D)   crural

54

A ____ fracture occurred in the hip area.
        A)   gluteal
        B)   lumbar
        C)   costal
        D)   coxal

55

A mental tumor could be one in the _____.
    A)   brain
    B)   thigh
    C)   jaw
    D)   leg

56

A cervical lesion could be on the uterus or _____.
    A)   neck
    B)   cheek
    C)   armpit
    D)   abdomen

57

A headache is an example of a _____ pain.
    A)   celiac
    B)   femoral
    C)   cephalic
    D)   gluteal

ANSWERS

1. B	17. A
2. D	18. B
3. C	19. A
4. B	20. C
5. B	21. D
6. C	22. B
7. C	23. A
8. B	24. C
9. C	25. B
10. D	26. C
11. B	27. A
12. A	28. D
13. B	29. C
14. C	30. B
15. D	31. A
16. C	32. B

33. C	46. B
34. C	47. C
35. A	48. D
36. B	49. D
37. B	50. D
38. C	51. D
39. D	52. D
40. A	53. B
41. B	54. D
42. B	55. C
43. D	56. A
44. C	57. C
45. C	

QUIZ 2

TRUE/ FALSE

1

The stethoscope is placed on the antecubital surface in order to assess a blood pressure.
- A) True
- B) False

2

Magnetic resonance imaging is a technique using radiation to view the internal structures.
- A) True
- B) False

3

Ultrasonography is a sensitive method of viewing the possibility of bone fractures.
- A) True
- B) False

4

A popliteal pulse would be felt above the femur.
- A) True
- B) False

5

Carbon dioxide can be a waste that must be eliminated from the body.
- A) True
- B) False

6

The property of responsiveness means that an organism will respond abnormally if stimulated.
- A) True
- B) False

7

All body structures must be associated with some type of functions and purposes.
   A)   True
   B)   False

8

If an organism displays the ability to reproduce itself at some time, including microorganisms, it is probably living.
   A)   True
   B)   False

9

Metabolism is a term, which can refer to the sum total of all chemical reactions in an organism.
   A)   True
   B)   False

10

An otic abnormality could be a deformed nasal septum.
   A)   True
   B)   False

11

Death is recognized as the absence of vital signs.
   A)   True
   B)   False

12

The skin is the part of the body that homeostatically maintains body temperature.
   A)   True
   B)   False

13

Normal body temperature, assessed below the tongue, is 20 degrees C.
- A)   True
- B)   False

14

Insulin decreases blood sugar levels while glucagon acts to increase blood glucose.
- A)   True
- B)   False

15

Diseases usually involve positive rather than negative feedback mechanisms.
- A)   True
- B)   False

16

Properties of an organ are usually considered to be the same as those of an organ system.
- A)   True
- B)   False

17

A bone cell would function the same whether it was alone or together with a group of similar cells.
- A)   True
- B)   False

18

The term parietal is used to name something on the surface of an organ.
- A)   True
- B)   False

19

The peritoneum is a type of abdominal membrane.
   A)   True
   B)   False

20

The parietal pleura is the membrane which covers the surface of each lung.
   A)   True
   B)   False

21

It is not correct to say that the lungs lie within the space called the pleural cavity.
   A)   True
   B)   False

22

The thymus gland lies on top of the heart in the mediastinum.
   A)   True
   B)   False

23

Serous fluid is usually protective and thick in consistency.
   A)   True
   B)   False

24

Nerve impulses usually have a relatively slow influence on target organs when compared to hormones.
   A)   True
   B)   False

25

The digestive system acts to bring foods into cells where they are broken down into usable forms.

    A)   True
    B)   False

26

The epididymis is part of the endocrine system.

    A)   True
    B)   False

27

The purpose of the reproductive system is for the continuation of the species.

    A)   True
    B)   False

28

In the anatomical position the palm of the hands face towards the back.

    A)   True
    B)   False

29

A peripheral wound could be located near the surface of the skin.

    A)   True
    B)   False

30

The term ipsilateral means on the opposite side.

    A)   True
    B)   False

31

Anterior can be used the same as ventral.

    A)   True

B)   False

32

The term transverse is identical to horizontal section.
    A)   True
    B)   False

33

The abdominal area could be divided into six regions or quadrants.
    A)   True
    B)   False

34

The term acromial indicates the elbow area.
    A)   True
    B)   False

ANSWERS

1. A
2. B - MRI uses magnetic forces to alter the spin of atoms and cause an electrical image to appear.
3. B - Ultrasound is best used to view soft structures such as fetuses.
4. B - The popliteal area is located behind the knee.
5. A - Carbon dioxide, like many other compounds, is essential for life, only the amount that is in excess is eliminated into the air during breathing, and therefore a waste
6. B - Responsiveness means that a cell or organism will make a response if stimulated.
7. A
8. A
9. A
10. B - The term otic refers to the ear.
11. A
12. B - The brain contains the control center (hypothalamus) which maintains temperature; the skin is an organ that responds to signals from the brain.
13. B - The average or normal oral temperature for adult humans is 37 degrees C (98.6 degreesF).
14. A
15. A

16. B - The properties of each level of organization are unique; as example, the beating of a heart outside of the body would not be able to be influenced by the same control mechanisms existing in the intact organism that affect heart function.

17. B - The function of individual cells (cytology) is uniquely different from a group of cells (histology) acting as a unit.

18. B - The term parietal means on the wall around the organ; visceral is the term for an organ.

19. A

20. B - The parietal pleura is the membrane directly on the surface of the thoracic cavity.

21. A

22. A

23. B - The serous fluid membranes are very wet and slippery to reduce friction.

24. B - The action and response of a nerve is almost immediate while chemical hormones require time to modify the metabolism of cells.

25. B - The activity of the digestive system occurs in the space surrounded by the lining of the digestive organs and is considered extracellular. Digestion occurs outside of cells; once substances enter cells they undergo processes referred to as metabolism.

26. B - The epididymis is a male reproductive structure.

27. A

28. B - The anatomical position requires that the palms face forward.

29. A

30. B - Ipsilateral means on the same side; contralateral refers to the opposite side.

31. A

32. A

33. B - The term quadrant implies four areas.

34. B - Acromial refers to a shoulder area.

1)   A (n) _____ muscle contraction changes tension, but remains the same length

    A.   Concentric
    B.   Isotonic
    C.   Physiologically fatigued
    D.   Isometric
    E.   Plyometric

2)   A cells plasma membrane would not contain

    A.   Phospholipids
    B.   Proteins
    C.   Cholesterol
    D.   Nucleic acids
    E.   All of the above are found in plasma membranes

3)   A codon is a three-base group of nucleotides that encodes a (n)

    A.   Phospholipid
    B.   Nucliec acid
    C.   Monosaccharide
    D.   Amino acid
    E.   Glycocalyx

4)   A developmental anatomist would be most likely to study

    A.   The effects of alcohol on the structure of the liver
    B.   The growth of the fetal nervous system in utero
    C.   Changes to muscle tissue as a result of exercise
    D.   How the adult brain responds to sleep deprivation
    E.   The process of bone repair following a break

5)   A joint cavity is found in

    A.   Synovial joints
    B.   Gomphoses
    C.   Syndesmoses

D. Both a and c

E. All of the above

6) A membrane potential can best be described as

A. An electrochemical gradient across a biological membrane
B. The ability of charged ion to carry an electrical signal in solution
C. The potential for a membrane to do work
D. The role of the plasma membrane in cell to cell recognition
E. The ability to transport vesicle to merge with the plasma membrane during exocytosis

7) A metabolic poison that inhibits the production of ATP most likely affects the

A. Mitochondria
B. Golgi apparatus
C. Ribosomes
D. Cytoskeleton
E. Lysosomes

8) A needle would pierce the epidermal layers of the forearm in which order?

A. Stratum granulosum, stratum corneum, straum basale, stratum spinosum
B. Stratum spinosum, stratum basale, stratum granulosum, stratum corneum
C. Stratum corneum, stratum spinosum, stratum granulosum, stratum basale
D. Stratum basale, stratum granulosum, stratum spinosum, stratum corneum
E. Stratum corneum, stratum granulosum, stratum spinosum, stratum basale

9) A patient has a ruptured appendix, into which activity would a surgeon cut

A. Abdominal
B. Thoracic
C. Vertebral
D. Cranial
E. Pleural

10) A person that has suffered a burn that resulted in red blistered skin on 10% of their epidermis would be categorized as _____ burn

A. 1st degree non critical burn

B.   2nd degree non critical burn
C.   2nd degree critical
D.   3rd degree non critical
E.   3rd degree critical

11)   A red blood cell placed in pure water would

A.   Swell
B.   Shrink initially, and then return to normal as equilibrium is reached
C.   Neither shrink nor swell
D.   Shrink only

12)   A strong acid _____ ionizes in water and results in a _____ pH.

A.   Partially, low
B.   Fully, high
C.   Partially, high
D.   Fully, low
E.   None of the above

13)   A structure that is composed of two or more tissues would be a (n)

A.   Organ
B.   Complex tissue
C.   Organelle
D.   Compound tissue
E.   Complex cell

14)   A thin layer of _____ provides cushioning at articulations

A.   Adipose tissue
B.   Hyaline cartilage
C.   Dense connective tissue
D.   Fibrocartilage
E.   Endosteum

15)   About 96% of the body is some combination of the following four elements:

A.   C, O, NA, H
B.   P, C, H, O

C.   N, C, O, K

D.   O, H, N, Ca

E.   H, O, C, N

16)   According to the size principle of multiple motor unit recruitment

     A.   Small motor units are most sensitive and recruited first
     B.   Large motor units are most sensitive and recruited first
     C.   Small motor units are most sensitive and recruited last
     D.   Large motor units are least sensitive and recruited last
     E.   Small motor units are least sensitive and recruited last

17)   Action potentials are propagated along the membrane primarily by

     A.   Leakage ion channels
     B.   Voltage gated ion channels
     C.   Mechanogated ion channels
     D.   Ligand gated ion channels

18)   After a fair skinned person spent the day at the beach with no sun screen which cell type is most likely to become highly active?

     A.   Keratinocyte
     B.   Melanocyte
     C.   Astrocyte
     D.   Matrix cell
     E.   Papillary cell

19)   After axonal injury, regeneration in peripheral nerves is guided by

     A.   Wallerian cells
     B.   Schwann cells
     C.   Dendrites
     D.   Golgi organs

20)   All preganglionic neurons of the ANS release acetylcholine

     A.   True
     B.   False

21) An atom is found to have 7 protons and 8 neutrons. The atom is:

    A.   Nitrogen with a mass number of 15
    B.   Carbon with a mass number of 8
    C.   Oxygen with a mass number of 8
    D.   Nitrogen with a mass number of 7
    E.   Oxygen with a mass number of 15

22) An example of an irregular bone would be

    A.   Thoracic vertebrae
    B.   Calcaneous
    C.   Sternum
    D.   Radius
    E.   Patella

23) An inhibitory postsynaptic potential (IPSP) is associated with

    A.   A change in sodium ion permeability
    B.   Hyperpolarization
    C.   Opening of voltage regulated channels
    D.   Lowering the threshold for an action potential to occur

24) Andergenic receptors are most likely found on

    A.   Effector organs of the sympathetic division
    B.   Post-ganglionic neurons in the parasympathetic division
    C.   The adrenal medulla
    D.   Preganglionic neurons in the sympathetic division

25) As a result of bone tissue response to mechanical stress (load) _____ occurs at sites of _____ stress.

    A.   Bone deposit, high
    B.   Bone resorption, high
    C.   Osteomalacia, high
    D.   Intramembranous ossification, low
    E.   Bony callus formation, continuous

26) At the intial stages of muscle activity ATP is first regenerated through the _____pathway

   A. Anaerobic glycolytic
   B. Creatine phosphate
   C. Cross bridge
   D. Lypolytic
   E. Aerobic respiratory

27) A_____ fracture is incomplete and common in the more flexible bones of children

   A. Compound
   B. Depression
   C. Green stick
   D. Supramembranous
   E. Catastrophic

28) Before puberty, long bone lengthens at a zone of cartilage called the

   A. Epiphyseal plate
   B. Articular cartilage
   C. Medullary cavity
   D. Spongy bone
   E. Primary ossification center

29) Broca's area _____

   A. Corresponds to Brodmann's area 8
   B. Is usually found in the right hemisphere
   C. Serves the recognition of complex objects
   D. Is considered a motor speech area

30) Bursae and tendon sheaths can best be described as _____

   A. Disks or wedges of connective tissue that cushion articular surfaces
   B. External layers of connective tissue that stabalize joints
   C. Bags of lubricant that reduce friction between the bones of a joint
   D. Extensions of the synovial membrane that allow passage of blood vessels and nerves to the interior of joints
   E. Sheet like indirect attachment for a skeletal muscle

31) Cancer that originates from the stratum spinosum is called

    A.   Basal cell carcinoma
    B.   Osteoesarcoma
    C.   Squamous cell carcinoma
    D.   Spinosal carcinoma
    E.   Melanoma

32) Cardiovascular effects of the sympathetic division include all except

    A.   Constriction of most blood vessels
    B.   Dilation of the vessels serving the skeletal muscles
    C.   Increase of heart rate and force
    D.   Dilation of the blood vessels serving the skin and digestive viscera

33) Cartilage is an example of _____ tissue

    A.   Stratified epithelial
    B.   Bone
    C.   Connective
    D.   Nervous
    E.   Alveolar

34) Cell junctions that promote the controlled exchange of materials between neighboring cells are called _____

    A.   Desmosomes
    B.   Gap junctions
    C.   Transmembrane proteins
    D.   Tight junctions
    E.   Secretory vesicles

35) Cells that exit the cell cycle are said to enter _____ phase

    A.   Terminal
    B.   G o
    C.   Stop
    D.   Mature
    E.   None of the above

36) Cerminous glands are located in the skin of the

    A.   Anogenital area
    B.   Ear canal
    C.   Mucous membranes
    D.   Nasal canals
    E.   Scalp

37)
Collections of nerve cell bodies outside the central nervous system are called

    A.   Nuclei
    B.   Nerves
    C.   Ganglia
    D.   Tracts

38) Compared to a solution with a pH of 6, a solution with a pH of 8 has:

    A.   100 times more H+
    B.   2 times more H+
    C.   100 times less H+
    D.   4 times less H+
    E.   1000 times less H+

39)
During _____ a protein is synthesized from mRNA

    A.   Transcription
    B.   Transgenesis
    C.   Translation
    D.   Elongation
    E.   RNA processing

40) Exocrine glandular tissue consists of _____ & _____ cells.

    A.   Secretory/duct
    B.   Cuboidal/ columnar
    C.   Basal/ apical
    D.   Dense/ loose
    E.   None of the above

41) Fast glycolytic muscle fibers tend to _____, compared to slow oxidative muscle fibers

    A.   Have a fast contraction cycle, but fatigue quickly
    B.   Have a slow contraction cycle but fatigue slowly
    C.   Have a fast contraction cycle, but fatigue slowly
    D.   Have a slow contraction cycle but fatigue quickly
    E.   None of the above

42) For the cross-bridge cycle to be initiated it is necessary for calcium to bind to

    A.   Actin
    B.   Myosin
    C.   Tropomyosin
    D.   Troponin
    E.   Acetylcholine

43) Freely moveable joints are classified as

    A.   Synthroses
    B.   Diarthroses
    C.   Condyles
    D.   Amphiarthroses
    E.   Gomphoses

44)
Functional classification of joints is based on movements allowed by the joint, are classified as slightly moveable joints

    A.   Synovial
    B.   Synathroses
    C.   Diathroses
    D.   Condyloses
    E.   Amphiarthoroses

45) Glycogen is important as a

    A.   Energy storage molecule in the liver
    B.   Plasma membrane marker for cell recognition (cell marker)
    C.   Monosaccharide important for cell growth

D. Structural element in the cytoskeleton
E. Backbone for building fat (triglyceride) molecules

46)
Histology is the study of

A. Tissues
B. Cells
C. DNA
D. Organ systems
E. The respiratory system

47) If the posterior portion of the neural tube failed to develop properly the

A. Spinal cord may be affected
B. Cranial nerves would not form
C. Hindbrain would not be present
D. Telencephalon would cease development

48) In a negative feedback mechanism

A. The effect is usually damaging to the body
B. The response of the effector is to enchance the original stimulus
C. The response of the effector is to end the original stimulus
D. Large changes in the state of the variable are stimulated
E. The negative feedback triggers a positive feedback loop

49) In one complete cycle of the sodium/potassium pump

A. 3 Na+ enter and 2 K+ exit the cell
B. 3 K+ enter and 2 Na+ exit the cell
C. 2 Na+ enter and 3 K+exit the cell
D. 2 K+ enter and 3 Na+ exit the cell
E. 3 Na+ enter and 3 K+ exit the cell

50) In response to vigorous activity/ exercise the blood vessels of the skin dilate (open) to allow greater blood flow to the surface of the body, this is an example of the integumentary system functioning in (as)

A. Cutaneous sensation

B.   Biological barrier
C.   Temperature regulation
D.   Excretion
E.   Energy source

51)   In the process of _____ cartilage forming cells in the perichondrium secrete new matrix against the external face of existing cartilage

A.   Intramembranous ossification
B.   Interstitial growth
C.   Calcification
D.   Bone remodeling
E.   Appositional growth

52)   In which phase of muscle contraction would you expect calcium to be returned to the sarcoplasmic reticulum?

A.   Latent phase
B.   Refractory phase
C.   Contractile phase
D.   Stimulation phase
E.   Relaxation phase

53)   Kyphosis (hunchback) results from exaggerated _____ curvature of the vertebral column

A.   Cervical
B.   Thoracic
C.   Lumbar
D.   Sacral
E.   Coccygeal

54)   Moving one's head back and forth in a "NO" fashion is an example of

A.   Flexion
B.   Extension
C.   Circumduction
D.   Rotation
E.   Opposition

55)   Muscle contraction always results in muscle shortening

A.   True
B.   False

56)   Muscle tone can best be described as

A.   The ability of the muscle to efficiently cause skeletal movements
B.   The feeling of well-being following exercise
C.   The state of sustained partial contraction
D.   The increase in capillary formation to support energy needs of active muscle
E.   None of the above

57)   Nerves that carry impulses toward the CNS only are

A.   Afferent nerves
B.   Efferent nerves
C.   Motor nerves
D.   Mixed nerves

58)   One of the defining characteristics of muscle tissue is contractility. Contractility can best be described as _____

A.   The ability to receive and respond to stimuli
B.   The ability to shorten forcibly when adequately stimulated
C.   The ability to be stretched or extended
D.   The ability of a muscle cell to recoil and resting length after being stretched

59)   Organic compounds both _____ & _____

A.   Carbon, oxygen
B.   Oxygen, hydrogen
C.   Hydrogen, carbon
D.   Oxygen, nitrogen
E.   Carbon, nitrogen

60)   Place the following in correct sequence from simplest to most complex
1. molecules
2. tissues
3. organ system
4. cells
5. organ

A.   1,2,4,3,5
B.   4,1,2,5,3
C.   1,4,2,5,3
D.   2,4,1,5,3
E.   3,5,2,4,1

61)   Plane joints allow nonaxial movement

A.   True
B.   False

62)   Pointing one's toes downward toward the ground is known as

A.   Dorsiflexion
B.   Plantar flexion
C.   Extension
D.   Inversion
E.   Opposition

63)   Potentially damaging stimuli that result in pain are selectively detected by

A.   Interceptors
B.   Photoreceptors
C.   Nociceptors
D.   Proprioceptors

64)   Preparing the body for the "flight-or fight" response is the role of the

A.   Sympathetic nervous system
B.   Cerebrum
C.   Parasympathetic nervous system
D.   Somatic nervous system

65)   Pressure, pain, and temperature receptors in the skin are

A.   Interoceptors
B.   Exteroceptors
C.   Proprioceptors
D.   Mechanoreceptors

66) Repolarization of sarcolemma following action potential is accomplished by

   A. Opening of voltage gated K+ channels
   B. Release of Ca2+ from the SR
   C. Release of acetylcholine from synaptic vesicles
   D. Regeneration of ATP after contraction
   E. The creatine phosphate pathway

67) Resistance exercise (weight lifting) is most likely to result in

   A. Increased size of fast glycolic muscle fibers (Correct Answer)
   B. Increased number of slow oxidative muscle fibers (Your Answer)
   C. Conversion of fast glycolytic fibers into slow oxidative fibers
   D. All of the above
   E. None of the above

68) Ribosomes located in/on the _____ synthesize proteins that are incorporated into the membrane or exported from the cell in vesicles

   A. Golgi apparatus
   B. Cytoplasm
   C. Endoplasmic reticulum
   D. Nuclear envelope
   E. Centriole

69) Ridges of tissue on the surface of the cerebral hemispheres are called

   A. Gyri
   B. Sulci
   C. Fissures
   D. Ganglia

70) RNA differs from DNA because RNA contains

   A. Thymine and no uracil
   B. Guanine and no cytocine
   C. Uracil and no thymine
   D. Adenine and no thymine
   E. Uracil and no cytocine

71) Saltatory conduction is made possible by

A.   The myelin sheath
B.   Large nerve fibers
C.   Diphasic impulses
D.   Erratic transmission of nerve impulses

72) Schwann cells are functionally similar to

A.   Ependymal cells
B.   Microglia
C.   Oligodendrocytes
D.   Astrocytes

73) Smooth muscle tissue is composed of two layers the ____ layer and the _____ layer.

A.   Fast, slow
B.   Active, inactive
C.   Sensitive, dense
D.   Longitudinal, circular
E.   Crossed, orthogonal

74) Sucrose is composed of one glucose and one fructose chemically bonded, so sucrose is considered a _____.

A.   Monosaccharide
B.   Dipeptide
C.   Polymer
D.   Disaccharide
E.   Polysaccharide

75) Sympathetic division stimulation causes

A.   A decreased blood glucose, increased GI peristalsis, and increased heart rate and blood pressure (Your Answer)
B.   Increase blood glucose, increased GI peristalsis, and decreased heart rate and blood pressure
C.   Increased blood glucose, decreased GI peristalsis, and increased heart rate and blood pressure

D. Decreased blood glucose, increased GI peristalsis, and decreased heart rate and blood pressure

Incorrect

76) Sympathetic responses generally are widespread because

A. Inactivation of ACh is fairly slow
B. NE and epinephrine are secreted into the blood as part of the sympathetic response
C. Preganglionic fibers are short
D. Preganglionc fibers are long

77) Synovial joints with a biaxial range of motion have the greatest range of motion

A. True
B. False

78) Temporal or wave summation of muscle twitch can best be described as

A. A wave of depolarization that travels down the sarcolemma
B. An increased rate of neural stimulation that leads to muscle twitch "piggy backing" before the muscle can fully relax
C. Process of sarcomere shortening resulting from the crossbridge cycle
D. Muscle adaptation that results from aerobic exercise
E. Increased motor unit recruitment that follows stronger neural signals

79) The anatomical position is used

A. Rarely because people seldom assume that position
B. As a standard reference for directional terms, regardless of the actual body position
C. Only by physicians during physical exams
D. Only when the body is lying down
E. None of the above

80) The arbor vitae refers to

A. Cerebellar gray matter
B. Cerebellar white matter
C. The pleatlike convolutions of the cerebellum
D. Flocculonodular nodes

81)
The axial skeleton includes all of the following

    A.   Sternum, sacrum, cranium
    B.   Tarsals, femur, humerous
    C.   Tibia, scapula, thoracic vertebrae
    D.   Cranium, vertebral column, pelvic girdle
    E.   None of the above

82)   The bonds in a water molecule can be best characterized as _____.

    A.   Ionic
    B.   Polar covalent
    C.   Non-polar covalent
    D.   Highly unstable
    E.   Semi-cationic

83)   The connective tissue sheath that surrounds a fascicle of a nerve fiber is the

    A.   Neurilema
    B.   Epineurium
    C.   Endoneurium
    D.   Perineurium

84)   The cranial sutures include the squamous, lambdoid, coronal, and

    A.   Deltoid
    B.   Sagital
    C.   Nasal
    D.   Mandibular
    E.   Ethmoid

85)   The division of anatomy that deals with large structures that are visible to the naked eye is called

    A.   Developmental anatomy
    B.   Gross anatomy
    C.   Histological anatomy
    D.   Coarse anatomy
    E.   Micro anatomy

86) The essential element of DNA that determines the order of amino acids in protein is

A. The sequence of the nucleotide bases
B. The regular alteration of sugar and phosphate molecules
C. The three-dimensional structure of the double helix
D. The ordered arrangement of the histones
E. The ratio between adenine and guanine

87) The femur is an example of a (n)

A. Long bone
B. Short bone
C. Flat bone
D. Intermediate bone
E. Irregular bone

88) The functional contractile unit of skeletal muscle is

A. Titin
B. The sacromere
C. The myofibril
D. The sacrolemma
E. None of the above

89) The functional unit of skeletal muscle is

A. Titin
B. The sarcomere
C. The myofibril
D. The sarcolemma
E. None of the above

90) The hypothalamus _____

A. Is the thermostat of the body because it regulates temperature
B. Is an important auditory and visual relay center
C. Has the pulvinar body as part of its structure
D. Mediates sensations

91) The linkage formed between amino acids in a protein is known as a (n) _____

    A.   Ionic bond
    B.   Peptide bond
    C.   Amino bond
    D.   Hydrogen bond
    E.   Polar bond

92) The main function of _____ is thermoregulation

    A.   Eccrine sweat glands
    B.   Aprocrine sweat glands
    C.   Mammary glands
    D.   Ceruminous glands
    E.   Pineal gland

93)
The major event of the S-phase of mitosis is

    A.   Synthesis of new nucleus
    B.   Condesing of the chromatin into chromosomes
    C.   Splitting of the cellular cytoplasm into two new cells
    D.   The chromosomes lining up at the "equator" of the cell
    E.   Replication of genomic DNA

94) The medullary cavity of a long bone is located in the _____and contains _____ which is_____

    A.   Diaphysis, red marrow, the site for hematopoiesis
    B.   Epiphysis, yellow marrow, used for osteogenesis
    C.   Spongy bone, red marrow, the site for immune response
    D.   Diaphysis, yellow marrow, adipose storage
    E.   Diaphysis, trabeculae, made of hydroxyapatite

95)
The most superficial layer of the dermis is the

    A.   Papillary layer
    B.   Stratum corneum
    C.   Reticular layer

D.   Stratum spinosum
E.   Stratum granulosum

96)   The movement of molecules or ions down their concentration gradient and across a biological membrane utilizing a transmembrane protein without the use of ATP is called

A.   Simple diffusion
B.   Facilitated diffusion
C.   Active transport
D.   Osmosis
E.   Complex diffusion

97)   The occipital bone of the skull is an example of a (n)

A.   Long bone
B.   Short bone
C.   Flat bone
D.   Intermediate bone
E.   Irregular bone

98)   The overall three-dimensional structure of one folded polypeptide (protein) is called its _____ structure.

A.   Primary
B.   Secondary
C.   Tertiary
D.   Quaternary
E.   Double helix

99)   The patellar "knee jerk" reflex is an example of a(n)

A.   Extensor thrust reflex
B.   Stress reflex
C.   Crossed extensor reflex
D.   Stretch reflex

100)   The period after an intial stimulus when a neuron is not sensitive to another stimulus is the _____.

A.   Resting period
B.   Repolarization

C. Depolarization
D. Absolute refractory period

101) The primary auditory cortex is located in the

A. Prefrontal lobe
B. Frontal lobe
C. Temporal lobe
D. Parietal lobe

102) The primary protein constituent of thick myofilaments is

A. Tropomyosin
B. Myosin
C. Actin
D. Troponin
E. Tubulin

103) The primary role of nervous tissue is to _____

A. Respond to stimuli and transmit electrical signals to other body regions
B. Pull on the skin and bones to create body movements
C. Provide cushioning and protection for vital organs
D. Function as a barrier

104) The principle that states that the structure and function of any bodily system are inseparable is known as the principle of

A. Symbiosis
B. Duality
C. Continuity
D. Sustainability
E. Complementarity

105) The process of bone remodling called bone resorption is accomplished by _____ in response to_____ Ca2+ levels in the blood

A. Osteoblasts, low
B. Osteoclasts, high
C. Osteoblasts, high
D. Osteoclasts, excessive
E. Osteoclasts, low

106) The region of the sarcolemma that carries an action potential into the deep interior of a muscle is called a

    A.   Neuromuscular junction
    B.   Myofibril
    C.   T- tubule
    D.   Aponeurosis
    E.   Motor end plate

107) The region of the sarcolemma that carries an action potential into the deep interior of a muscle is called a

    A.   Neuromuscular junction
    B.   Terminal cisterna
    C.   T-tubule
    D.   Aponeruosis
    E.   Motor end plate

108) The rib cage contains ___true ribs,___ false ribs, and _____ floating ribs

    A.   7, 3, 2
    B.   8, 2, 3
    C.   6, 4, 3
    D.   10, 1, 2
    E.   9, 4, 4

109) The role of cholestrol in the plasma membrane is to

    A.   Prevent excess sodium from entering the cell
    B.   Act as an "identification tag" for neighboring cells
    C.   Import glucose molecules
    D.   Stabalize and increase the fluidity of the membrane
    E.   Increase surface area to aid absorption

110) The sarcoplasmic reticulum stores what cation?

    A.   Potassium
    B.   Sodium

C. Phosphate
D. Calcium
E. Magnesium

111) The sliding filament model of contraction involves

A. Actin and myosin filaments sliding past each other while partially overlapping
B. The shortening of thick filaments so that each thin filament slides past it
C. Actin being broken down during each contraction and replaced while resting
D. Actin heads binding to ATP and sliding the myosin filaments inward
E. Actin and myosin filaments getting shorter, but not sliding past each other

112) The sodium/potassium pump is an example of

A. Simple diffusion
B. Facilitated diffusion
C. Osmosis
D. Active transport
E. Receptor mediated endocytosis

113) The stratum basale of the epidermis can best be described as

A. Playing a major role in water proofing the skin
B. Simple epithelium with an excretory function
C. Primarily immune system cells
D. Storage cell for subcutaneous fat
E. Single layer of mitotically active cells

114) The stratum lucidum is found

A. Just deep to the papillary layer
B. Within the areolar tissue of the dermal layer
C. Only in thick skin
D. More in females than males
E. All of the above

115) The structure in compact bone that runs perpendicular (right angle) to connect adjacent osteons is called _____.

A. Volkmann's canal

B. Circumferential lamellae
C. Haversian canal
D. Lacunae
E. Trabeculae

116) The subarachnoid space lies between what two layers of meninges?

A. Arachnoid and epidura
B. Arachnoid and pia
C. Arachnoid and dura
D. Dura and epidura

117) The subatomic particle that determines what the specific element is:

A. Electron
B. Proton
C. Isotope
D. Neutron
E. Lepton

118) The thalamus and the hypothalamus are both located

A. In the cerebrum
B. In the diencephalon
C. Next to the medula
D. Posterior to the cerebellum

119) The three primary element of the cytoskeleton are microfilaments, intermediate filaments and

A. Centrioles
B. Nuclear pores
C. Microtubules
D. Connexons
E. Fibrocytes

120) The two layers of an articular capsule of a synovial joint are _____ and_____.

A. Intervening pad, periosteum
B. Fibrous capsule, synovial membrane

C. Synovial membrane, bursa
D. Fibrous capsule, fatty pad
E. None of the above

121) The _____ bone is an example of a facial bone

A. Zygomatic
C. Lamboid
D. Temporal
E. Occipital

122) The _____ give an osteon a structure resembling tree rings

A. Canaliculi
B. Lamellae
C. Central canal
D. Trabeculae
E. Volkmanns canal

123) The _____ system eliminates nitrogenous waste and regulates water and electrolyte balance

A. Digestive
B. Excretory
C. Respiratory
D. Cardiovascular
E. Endocrine

124)
These cells primarily function as part of the integuments role as a biological barrier

A. Langerhans (dendritic) cells
B. Melanocytes
C. Merkel
D. Arrector pili
E. Alpha cells

125) The _____ is an example of a hinge joint

A. Shoulder

B. Wrist
C. Elbow
D. Temporomandibular
E. None of the above

126) The_____joint is an example of a ball and socket joint

A. Shoulder
B. Wrist
C. Elbow
D. Temporomandibular
E. None of the above

127) Virtually all chemical reactions in our body are catalized (sped up) by

A. Salts
B. Enzymes
C. Phospholipids
D. Polysaccharides
E. Electrolytes

128) The primary role of the biological pigment melanin is

A. Cutaneous stretch sensation
B. Protect DNA from UV damage
C. Activate immune cells in response to microorganisms
D. Aid in tissue repair after mechanical stress/ damage
E. None of the above

129) _____ muscle tissue is striated, branched and has intercalated disks

A. Skeletal
B. Voluntary
C. Involuntary
D. Cardiac
E. Smooth

130) _____ adhere neighboring cells together so that no fluids or solutes may pass between the cells

A. Tight junctions

B.   Connexons
C.   Keratin
D.   Desmosomes
E.   Gap junctions

131)   _____ epithelium appears to have two or three layers of cells, but all the cells are in contact with the basement membrane

   A.   Simple squamous
   B.   Complex
   C.   Stratified
   D.   Cuboidal
   E.   Pseudostratified

132)   _____consists of a layer of spongy bone sandwiched between two layers of compact bone

   A.   Periosteum
   B.   Flat bone
   C.   Diaphysis
   D.   Interstitial lamellae
   E.   Hyaline cartilage

133)
Wolfs law is concerned with _____

   A.   Calcium homeostasis
   B.   The thickness and strength of bone being determined by mechanical and gravitational forces
   C.   The electrical charge in the bone surface
   D.   The rate of bone repair following a fracture
   E.   The strength to weight ratio of bone tissue determined by the relative composition of organic and inorganic components

134)   Which type of muscle tissue would be found in the walls of arteries?

   A.   Striated muscle
   B.   Skeletal muscle
   C.   Caridac muscle
   D.   Smooth muscle
   E.   None of the above

135) Which structure of the integumentary system would most likely respond to a sudden drop in temperature?

    A.   Eccrine glands
    B.   Arrector pili
    C.   Ceruminous glands
    D.   Pacinian corpuscle
    E.   Merkel disk

136) Which statement best describes connective tissue?

    A.   Usually contains large amounts of extracellular matrix
    B.   Primary concerned with secretion
    C.   Usually lines a body cavity or covers an organ
    D.   Typically arranged in a single cell layer
    E.   Mostly functions to signal information to other tissues

137) Which of these nonmetals is not listed with the number of covalent bonds it naturally forms?

    A.   O oxygen 2
    B.   C carbon 3
    C.   N nitrogen 3
    D.   H hydrogen 1
    E.   Na sodium 2

138) Which of the following systems is dependent on the cardiovascular system for its function?

    A.   Digestive system
    B.   Nervous system
    C.   Skeletal system
    D.   Integumentary system
    E.   All of the above

139) Which of the following is true concerning the atomic nucleus?

    A.   Contains the mass of the atom
    B.   Contains the particle that create chemical bonds
    C.   Contains negatively charged particles
    D.   Its mass is constantly changing

E.   None of the above

140) Which of the following is not a functional characteristic of life?

    A.   Movement
    B.   Responsiveness to external stimuli
    C.   Maintenance of external boundary
    D.   Decay
    E.   Reproduction

141) Which of the following is not a characteristic of epithelial tissue

    A.   Exhibits polarity
    B.   Supported by connective tissue
    C.   Highly vascular (supplied with blood vessels)
    D.   Innervated (supplied by nerve fibers)
    E.   Highly regenerative

142) Which of the following is an example of a lipid?

    A.   Amino acid
    B.   Cholesterol
    C.   Enzymes
    D.   Glycogen
    E.   Tryptophan

143) Which of the following is a principle of the fluid mosaic model of cell membrane structure?

    A.   The cell membrane is solid at room temperature thus protecting the cell
    B.   Membrane proteins "float" within the lipid bilayer creating a constantly changing mosaic pattern
    C.   Membrane proteins transport fluids from the interior to the exterior of the cell
    D.   The phospholipids that compose the membrane are tightly attached to each other to prevent fluid loss
    E.   None of the above

144) Which of the following epidermal glands produces a milky sweat that tends to become odoriferous over time?

A. Sebaceous
B. Eccrine
C. Merkel
D. Aprocrine
E. Axillary

145) Which of the following elements is most likely to form an ionic bond with potassium (atomic symbol K)?

A. Carbon
B. Oxygen
C. Sodium
D. Chlorine
E. Nitrogen

146)
Which is not essential for survival

A. Water
B. Oxygen
C. Nutrients
D. Light
E. None of the above

147)
Which element is matched with the correct number of valence electrons

A. Carbon, 5
B. Sodium, 1
C. Oxygen, 3
D. Nitrogen, 2
E. Chlorine, 6

148) What chemical is stored in the synaptic vesicles of a motor neuron?

A. potassium
B. Sodium
C. ATP
D. Calcium
E. Acetylcholine

149) What is the direct role of ATP hydrolysis in skeletal muscle contraction?

     A.   Promotes a shift of tropomyosin, exposing myosin binding sites on actin
     B.   Opens calcium channels in the sarcoplasmic reticulum
     C.   Return the myosin head to the high energy "cocked" position
     D.   Allows the myosin to form cross bridges with the actin filament
     E.   None of the above

150) What is aponeurosis?

     A.   A sheet like extension of connective tissue that provides indirect attachment for muscles to bone
     B.   A wispy sheath of connective tissue that surround each individual muscle fiber
     C.   An "overcoat" of dense irregular connective tissue that surrounds the whole muscle
     D.   Granule of stored glycogen that provides glucose during muscle activity
     E.   A rod like bundle of contractile filaments

151) What is acetylchoinesterase?

     A.   An enzyme that breaks down acetylcholine
     B.   Signaling molecule that initiates contraction
     C.   Protein that blocks the myosin binding site on actin filaments
     D.   The control center for excitation contraction coupling
     E.   None of the above

152) What are ciliated CNS neuroglia that play an active role in moving the cerebrospinal fluid called?

     A.   Ependymal cells
     B.   Schwann cells
     C.   Oligodendrocytes
     D.   Astrocytes

153) Which of the following is false or incorrect?

     A.   An excitatory postsynaptic potential occurs if the excitatory effect is greater than the inhibitory effect but less than threshold

B.   A nerve impulse occurs if the excitatory and inhibitory effects are equal
C.   An inhibitory postsynaptic potential occurs if the inhibitory effect is greater than the excitatory, causing hyperpolarization of the membrane

154) Which of the following is not true of graded potentials

A.   They are short lived
B.   They can form on receptor endings
C.   They increase amplitude as they move away from the stimulus point
D.   They can be called postsynaptic potentials

155) Which of the following is not a special characteristic of neurons?

A.   They conduct impulses
B.   They have extreme longevity
C.   They are mitotic
D.   They have an exceptionally high metabolic rate

156) Which fissure separates the cerebral hemispheres?

A.   Central fissure
B.   Longitudinal fissure
C.   Parieto-occipital fissure
D.   Lateral fissure

157)
Which statement correctly describes an anatomical feature of the ANS

A.   The parasympathetic division has long post-ganglionic neurons
B.   The sympathetic division exits the CNS in the thoraco-lumbar region of the spinal chord
C.   The parasympathetic division exits the CNS through the lumbar and sacral regions of the spinal chord
D.   The sympathetic post-ganglionic neurons are heavily mylenated

ANSWERS

	5. A	10. B
1. D	6. A	11. A
2. D	7. A	12. D
3. D	8. E	13. A
4. B	9. A	14. B

15. E	60. C		103.	A
16. A	61. A		104.	E
17. B	62. B		105.	E
18. B	63. C		106.	C
19. B	64. A		107.	C
20. A	65. B		108.	A
21. A	66. A		109.	D
22. A	67. A		110.	D
23. B	68. C		111.	A
24. A	69. A		112.	D
25. A	70. C		113.	E
26. B	71. A		114.	C
27. C	72. C		115.	A
28. A	73. D		116.	B
29. D	74. D		117.	B
30. C	75. C		118.	B
31. C	76. B		119.	C
32. D	77. B		120.	B
33. C	78. B		121.	A
34. B	79. B		122.	B
35. B	80. B		123.	B
36. B	81. A		124.	A
37. C	82. B		125.	C
38. C	83. D		126.	A
39. C	84. B		127.	B
40. A	85. B		128.	B
41. B	86. A		129.	D
42. D	87. A		130.	A
43. B	88. B		131.	E
44. E	89. B		132.	D
45. A	90. A		133.	B
46. A	91. B		134.	D
47. A	92. A		135.	B
48. C	93. E		136.	A
49. D	94. D		137.	B
50. C	95. A		138.	E
51. E	96. B		139.	A
52. E	97. C		140.	D
53. B	98. C		141.	C
54. D	99. D		142.	C
55. B			143.	B
56. C			144.	D
57. A	100.	D	145.	D
58. B	101.	C	146.	D
59. C	102.	B	147.	B

148. E
149. C
150. A
151. A
152. A
153. B
154. C
155. C
156. B
157. B

1. A decrease in blood osmolality results in
   a) increased ADH secretion
   b) increased permeability of the collecting ducts to H_2O
   c) decreased urine osmolarity
   d) decreased urine output
2. The permeability of the walls of the distal convoluted tubules are regulated by
   a) the amount of H_2O
   b) the concentration of salts
   c) vasopressin
   d) the adrenals
   e) the thymus

3. If blood becomes hypertonic, the kidney will
   a) secrete more ADH
   b) excrete more H_2O
   c) decrease filtration rate
   d) excrete smaller volumes of concentrated urine
   e) increase filtration rate
4. H^+ ions are not able to lower blood pH because they are:
   a) removed by carbonic anhydrase
   b) bound to H_2O
   c) bound to hemoglobin
   d) removed by diffusion
   e) bound to CO_2
5. All of the following enzymes are involved in the digestion of food, EXCEPT
   a) pepsin
   b) trypsin
   c) maltase
   d) amylase
   e) ligase
6. Exocrine gastric product that combines with B_{12} for absorption in the small intestine:
   a) pepsin
   b) HCl
   c) mucus
   d) Intrinsic Factor
   e) trypsin
7. The most abundant proteins in blood plasma are:
   a) globulins
   b) transport proteins
   c) albumins
   d) lipoproteins

8. The alveolar respiratory membrane consists mainly of
    a) pseudostratified ciliated columnar epithelium
    b) moist cuboidal epithelium
    c) simple squamous epithelium
    d) ciliated squamous epithelium
    e) surfactant cells
9. Luteinizing hormone (LH) and follicule stimulating hormone (FSH) are secreted by which gland?
    a) anterior pituitary
    b) posterior pituitary
    c) thyroid
    d) adrenal medulla
    e) adrenal cortex
10. Ovum and follicle development is stimulated by
    a) increased FSH production
    b) low estrogen levels
    c) high estrogen levels
    d) high progesterone levels
    e) low progesterone levels

11. During the menstrual cycle, peak levels of estrogen and luteinizing hormone (LH) are associated with
    a) the flow phase
    b) the early part of the follicular phase
    c) the latter part of the follicular phase
    d) the early part of the luteal phase
    e) the latter part of the luteal phase
12. During the proliferative phase of the female reproductive cycle, the pituitary increases secretion of
    a) luteinizing hormone (LH)
    b) follicle stimulating hormone (FSH)
    c) progesterone
    d) estrogen
    e) adrenocorticotropic hormone (ACH)
13. What does NOT occur immediately after fertilization?
    a) a sperm enters the outer membrane of the egg
    b) cytoplasmic substances in the fertilized egg become rearranged
    c) the genetic material of the sperm and egg combine
    d) cleavage occurs
    e) none of the above
14. The stage during development in which there is a hallow ball of cells is called
    a) blastulation
    b) morulation
    c) the isolecithal stage
    d) gastrulation

e) ovulation

15. What is the total volume of air inhaled per minute if a person has a tidal volume of 600 ml and breathes at a rate of 11 cycles per minute?
    a) 55 mL
    b) 66 mL
    c) 250 mL
    d) 1,000 mL
    e) 6,600 mL

16. The enzymatic breakdown of large molecules into their basic building blocks is called
    a) absorption
    b) secretion
    c) mechanical digestion
    d) chemical digestion

17. The outer layer of the digestive tract is known as the
    a) serosa
    b) mucosa
    c) submucosa
    d) muscularis

18. Double sheets of peritoneum that provide support and stability for the organs in the peritoneal cavity
    a) mediastina
    b) mucous membranes
    c) omenta
    d) mesenteries

19. A branch of the portal vein, hepatic artery, and tributary of the bile duct form
    a) a liver lobule
    b) the sinusoids
    c) a portal area
    d) the hepatic duct
    e) the pancreatic duct

20. Most of the digestive tract is lined by ____ epithelium
    a) pseudostratified ciliated columnar
    b) cuboidal
    c) stratified squamous
    d) simple
    e) simple columnar

21. Regional movements that occur in the small intestine and function to churn and fragment the digestive material are called
    a) segmentation
    b) pendular movements
    c) peristalsis

d) mass movements

22. Bile released from the gallbladder into the duodenum occurs only under the stimulation of
    a) cholecystokinin
    b) secretin
    c) gastrin
    d) enterpeptidase

23. The major functions of the large intestine are all of the following, except
    a) reabsorption of H_2O and compaction of feces
    b) absorption of vitamins liberated by bacterial action
    c) segmentation and compaction of feces
    d) storage of fecal matter

24. Vitamins generated by bacteria in the colon are
    a) A, D, and E
    b) B complexes and vitamin C
    c) vitamin E, biotin, and pantothenic acid
    d) niacin, thiamine, and riboflavin
    e) a and d only

25. The final enzymatic steps in the digestive process are accomplished by
    a) enzymes secreted by the stomach
    b) the action of bile from the gallbladder
    c) brush border enzymes of the intestinal microvilli
    d) the assistance of H_2CO_3 molecules
    e) a and c

26. The following all occur during defecation, except
    a) relaxation of the anal sphincter while the external anal sphincter contracts
    b) peristaltic contractions in the colon and rectum initiated by stretch muscles
    c) activation of stretch receptors in the rectal wall via activation of parasympathetic centers in the sacral region of the spinal cord

27. Increased parasympathetic stimulation of the intestine would result in
    a) decreased mobility and secretion processes
    b) decreased sensitivity of local reflexes
    c) decreased segmentation
    d) none of the above
    e) a and c only

28. A drop in pH below 4.5 in the duodenum stimulates the secretion of
    a) secretin
    b) cholecystokinin
    c) gastrin, secretin, and pantothenic acid
    d) all of the above
    e) b and c only

29. Catabolism refers to
    a) the breakdown of a nutrient pool

b) localized destruction of a nutrients
c) the breakdown of synthetic substrates
d) the breakdown of organic substrates
e) localized breakdown of glycogen

30. The breakdown of glucose into pyruvate is an _____ process
    a) anaerobic
    b) aerobic
    c) oxidative
    d) a and c
    e) b and c

31. The process that produces more than 90% of the ATP used by our cells is
    a) glycolysis
    b) the citric acid cycle
    c) the Krebs cycle
    d) oxidative phosphorylation
    e) substrate-level phosphorylation

32. The citric acid cycle must turn ___ times to completely metabolize the pyruvate produced from one glucose molecule
    a) 11
    b) 2
    c) 3
    d) 8
    e) 4

33. The largest metabolic reserves for the average adult are stored as
    a) carbohydrates
    b) fatty acids
    c) amino acids
    d) triglycerides
    e) albumin

34. The vitamins generally associated with vitamin toxicity are
    a) fat-soluble vitamins
    b) water-soluble vitamins
    c) B complex vitamins
    d) vitamins C and B_{12}

35. When blood levels of glucose, amino acids, and insulin are high and glycogenesis is occurring in the liver, the body is the _____ state.
    a) fasting
    b) metabolic state
    c) absorptive
    d) post absorptive

36. The glomerular filtration rate is regulated by all of the following, except
    a) auto regulation
    b) sympathetic neural control
    c) cardiac output
    d) angiotensin II
    e) b and c
37. The process of urine formation involves all of the following, except
    a) filtration of plasma
    b) H_2O reabsorption
    c) reabsorption of certain solutes
    d) secretion of wastes
    e) secretion of lipoprotein and glucose molecules

38. The distal convoluted tubule is an important site for
    a) active secretion of ions
    b) active secretion of acids
    c) selective reabsorption of Na^+ ions from the tubular fluid
    d) all of the above
    e) none of the above
39. Changing the diameters of the afferent and efferent arterioles to alter the GFR in an example of ____ regulation.
    a) hormonal
    b) autonomic
    c) auto regulation
    d) all of the above
    e) a and b only
40. When the renal threshold for a substance exceeds its tubular maximum,
    a) more of the substance will be filtered
    b) less of the substance will be filtered
    c) more of the substance will be secreted
    d) more of the substance will appear in the urine

41. Sympathetic activation of nerve fibers in the nephron causes all of these, except
    a) the regulation of glomerular blood flow and pressure
    b) the stimulation of renin release from the JGC
    c) the direct stimulation of H_2O and Na^+ reabsorption
    d) all of these occur
    e) b and c

42. Na^+ reabsorption in the DCT and the cortical portion of the collecting system is accelerated by the secretion of
    a) ADH
    b) renin
    c) aldosterone
    d) erythropoietin

43. Which of the following contribute to the formation of a hyperosmotic environment in the medulla of the kidney?
     a) impermeability of the ascending limb of the loop of Henle
     b) effects of ADH on water permeability of the ascending loop of Henle
     c) cotransport of Na^+, K^+, and Cl^- out of the ascending loop of Henle
     d) both a and c
     e) both b and c
44. At which of these sites is the osmolarity concentration at the lowest?
     a) glomerular capillary
     b) proximal convoluted tubule
     c) bottom of the loop of Henle
     d) initial section of the distal convoluted tubule
     e) section of the distal convoluted tubule directly before the collecting duct
45. A decrease in blood osmolarity results in which of these?
     a) increased ADH secretion
     b) increased permeability of the collecting ducts to H_2O
     c) decreased urine osmolarity
     d) decreased urine output
     e) all of the above

46. The amount of a substance that passes through the filtration membrane into the nephron per minute is the
     a) renal plasma flow
     b) tubular load
     c) plasma clearance
     d) tubular maximum
     e) renal threshold

47. H_2O leaves the nephron by
     a) active transport
     b) filtration
     c) osmosis
     d) facilitated diffusion
     e) cotransport
48. Surfactant
     a) protects the surface of the lungs
     b) phagocytizes into smaller particles
     c) replaces mucus in the alveoli
     d) helps prevent the alveoli from collapsing
     e) indicates abnormal lung tissue

49. Air moves into the lungs because
     a) the gas pressure in the lungs is less than atmospheric pressure
     b) the volume of the lungs decreases with inspiration

c) contraction of the diaphragm decreases the volume of the thoracic cavity
d) the intercostal nerves signals the respiratory center to initiate active expansion of the lungs
50. When the diaphragm and external intercostal muscles contract,
    a) exhalation occurs
    b) intrapulmonary pressure increases
    c) intrapleural pressure decreases
    d) lung volume decreases
    e) the thoracic cavity expands

ANSWERS

1. C	27. D
2. C	28. A
3. D	29. D
4. C	30. D
5. E	31. D
6. D	32. B
7. C	33. D
8. C	34. A
9. A	35. C
10. A	36. C
11. C	37. E
12. B	38. D
13. E	39. D
14. A	40. D
15. E	41. D
16. D	42. C
17. A	43. C
18. D	44. D
19. C	45. B
20. E	46. B
21. A	47. C
22. A	48. D
23. C	49. A
24. C	50. C
25. C	
26. A	

Quiz 5

1.Which of the following is NOT a function of skin?
a) respiration
b) excretion
c) sensation
d) thermoregulation

2.Which pigment is responsible for a tan's brown color?
a) melanin
b) carotene
c) hemoglobin
d) bile

3.What is redness of the skin called?
a) pallor
b) carotenemia
c) erythema
d) jaundice
e) eczema

4.skin sensitivity characterized by intense itching & inflammation:
a) urticaria
b) pruritis
c) shingles
d) psoriasis
e) eczema

5.a viral infection that follows nerve pathways, producing small lesions on the overlying skin:
a) urticaria
b) pruritis
c) shingles
d) psoriasis
e) eczema

6.severe itching of the skin:
a) urticaria
b) pruritis
c) shingles

d) psoriasis
e) eczema

7.allergic reaction characterized by the appearance of wheals:
a) urticaria
b) pruritis
c) shingles
d) psoriasis
e) eczema

8.chronic skin disease characterized by red flat areas covered with silvery scales:
a) urticaria
b) pruritis
c) shingles
d) psoriasis
e) eczema

9.the epidermis is ----------- to the dermis.
a) superfiicial
b) deep
c) lateral
d) medial

10.acne is an infection of which type of gland?
a) sudoriferous
b) sebaceous
c) ceruminous
d) meibomian

11.what is the medical term for baldness?
a) alopecia
b) pemphigus
c) verruca
d) dermatitis

12.which skin disorder is caused by an accumulation of bile pigment in the blood?
a) pallor
b) cyanosis
c) jaundice
d) carotenemia

13.which are affected in basal cell & squamous cell carcinomas?

a) epidermal cells
b) dermal cells
c) melanocytes
d) adipocytes

14.Which protein makes up a major component of bone matrix?
a) keratin
b) collagen
c) melanin
d) calcium

15.Where does bone growth occur in children?
a) center of bone shafts
b) epiphyseal plates
c) medullary cavities
d) epiphyseal lines

16.Which bone forms the back & parts of the base of the skull?
a) parietal bone
b) temporal bone
c) occipital bone
d) sphenoid bone

17.Which of the following bones is found in the shoulder girdle?
a) sternum
b) humerus
c) scapula
d) ulna

18.Freely movable joints are also called
a) fibrous joints
b) cartilaginous joints
c) diarthroses
d) amphiarthroses

19..A rounded bony projection
a) condyle
b) foramen
c) fossa
d) sinus
e) spine

20.A sharp bony prominence
a) condyle
b) foramen
c) fossa
d) sinus
e) spine

21.A hole through a bone
a) condyle
b) foramen
c) fossa
d) sinus
e) spine

22.A bony depression
a) condyle
b) foramen
c) fossa
d) sinus
e) spine

23.An air-filled bony cavity
a) condyle
b) foramen
c) fossa
d) sinus
e) spine

24.Which bone contains the mastoid process?
a) occipital bone
b) femur
c) temporal bone
d) humerus

25.What is an abnormal exaggeration of the thoracic curve called?
a) kyphosis
b) lordosis
c) osteitis deformans
d) Pott disease

26.Which injury is associated with multiple fracture lines & splintered or crushed bone?
a) open fracture
b) impacted fracture
c) comminuted fracture
d) greenstick fracture

27.Which joint is freely movable?
a) arthrotic
b) amphiarthrotic
c) diathrotic
d) synarthrotic

28.What kind of synovial joint is the hip?
a) gliding
b) hinge
c) pivot
d) ball & socket

29.which type of muscle tissue is striated & involuntary?
a) cardiac
b) intercalated
c) smooth
d) skeletal

30.a single neuron & all the muscle fibers it stimulates comprise:
a) motor end plate
b) motor unit
c) neuromuscular junction
d) synapse

31.the 2 filaments that form cross-bridges are
a) actin & troponin
b) tropomyosin & myosin
c) actin & myosin
d) troponin & tropomyosin

32.which muscle cell compound stores oxygen?
a) creatine phosphate
b) glycogen
c) hemoglobin

d) myoglobin

33.in anatomic lever systems, the fulcrum is the
a) bone
b) bursa
c) insertion
d) joint

34.an antagonist to the gastronemius is the
a) gracilis
b) sartorius
c) soleus
d) tibialis anterior

35.from superficial to deep the correct order of muscle structure is
a) deep fascia, epimysium, perimysium, & endomysium
b) epimysium, perimysium, endomysium & deep fascia
c) deep fascia, endomysium, perimysium, & epimysium
d) endomysium, perimysium, epimysium & deep fascia

36.what is the function of calcium ions in skeletal muscle contractions?
a) bind to receptors on the motor end plate to stimulate muscle contraction
b) cause a pH change in the cytoplasm to trigger muscle contraction
c) bind to the myosin-binding sites on actin so that myosin will have something to attach to
d) bind to regulatory proteins so that the myosin binding sites on the actin can be exposed

37.which structure is a broad flat extension that attaches muscle to bone?
a) tendon
b) fascicle
c) aponeurosis
d) motor end plate

38.what are seizures & convulsions examples of?
a) strains
b) fibrositis
c) myositis
d) spasms

ANSWERS

1. d) thermoregulation
2. a) melanin
3. b) erythema
4. eczema
5. c) shingles
6. b) pruritis
7. a) urticaria
8. d) psoriasis
9. a) superficial
10. b) sebaceous
11. a) alopecia
12. c) jaundice
13. a) epidermal cells
14. b) collagen
15. b) epiphyseal plates
16. c) occipital bone
17. c) scapula
18. c) diarthroses
19. a) condyle
20. e) spine
21. b) foramen
22. c) fossa
23. d) sinus
24. c) temporal bone
25. a) kyphosis
26. c) comminuted
27. c) diathrotic
28. d) ball-and-socket
29. a) cardiac
30. a) motor end plate
31. c) actin and myosin
32. d) myoglobin
33. d) joint
34. d) tibialis anterior
35. a) deep fascia, epimysium, perimysium, and endomysium
36. d) bind to regulatory proteins so that the myosin binding sites on the actin can be exposed
37. (c) aponeurosis
38. d) spasms

1. Blood leaves the right ventricle by passing through the
a) Aortic valve
b) Pulmonary valve
c) Mitral valve
d) Tricuspid valve
e) Bicuspid valve

Answer: b) pulmonary valve

2. Blood returning to the heart from the systemic circuit first enters the
a) Right atrium
b) Right ventricle
c) Left atrium
d) Left ventricle
e) conus arteriosus

answer: a) right atrium

3. The region in the thoracic cavity occupied by the heart, great vessels, thymus, esophagus, and trachea called the
a) pleural space.
b) pericardial space
c) mediastinum
d) cardiac notch
e) ventral cavity

answer: c) mediastinum

4. The visceral pericardium is the same as the
a) mediastinum
b) parietal pericardium
c) epicardium
d) myocardium
e) endocardium

answer: c) epicardium

5. Most of the middle layer in the heart wall is composed of
a) cardiac muscle cells
b) chondrocytes
c) epitheliocytes
d) fibrocytes

e) smooth muscle cells

answer: a) cardiac muscle cells

6. The left vertricle pumps blood to the
a) lungs
b) right ventricle
c) right atrium
d) aorta
e) pulmonary circuit

answer: d) aorta

7. coronary veins empty into the
a) left atrium
b) left ventricle
c) right atrium
d) right ventricle
e) conus arteriosus

answer: c) right atrium

8. The pulmonary semilunar valve prevents backward flow into the
a) arota
b) pulmonary trunk
c) pulmonary veins
d) right ventricle
e) left atrium

answer: d) right ventricle

9. The function of an atrium is to
a) collect blood
b) pump blood to the lungs
c) pump blood to the systemic circuit
d) pump blood to the ventricle
e) collect blood them pump it to the ventricle

answer: e) collect blood then pump it to the ventricle

10. The following is a list of vessels and structure that are associated with the heart.
1. right atrium
2. left atrium
3. right ventricle
4. left ventricle

5. venae cava
6. aorta
7. pulmonary trunk
8. pulmonary veins
what is the correct order for the flow of blood entering from the systemic circulation?
a) 1, 2,7,8,3,4,6,5
b) 1, 7,3,8,2,4,6,5
c) 5, 1,3,7,8,2,4,6
d) 5, 3,1,7,8,4,2,6
e) 5, 1,3,8,7,2,4,6

answer: c) 5, 1,3,7,8,2,4,6

11. The pulmonary arteries carry blood to the
a) heart
b) lungs
c) brain
d) intestines
e) liver

answer: b) lungs

12. The long plateau of the cardiac muscle action potential is due to
a) movement of fewer sodium ions across the cell membrane
b) calcium channels remaining open
c) increased membrane permeability to potassium ion
d) decrease in the amount of calcium diffusing across the membrane
e) increased membrane permeability to sodium ions.

answer: b) calcium channels remaining open

13. In cardiac muscle
a) calcium ions are not released from the sarcoplasmic reticulum
b) calcium ions do not bind to troponin molecules
c) calcium ions play no role in the process of contraction
d) about 20 percent of the calcium ion required for contraction comes from outside the cell
e) calcium ions play an important role in repolarizing the membrane after the depolarization phase

answer: d) about 20 percent of the calcium ion required for contraction comes from outside the cell

14. The following are structural components of the conducting system of the heart
1. Purkinje fibers
2. AV bundle

3. AV node
4. SA node
5. bundle branches
The sequence in which excitation would move through this system is
a) 1, 4,3,2,5
b) 3, 2,4,5,1
c) 3, 5,4,2,1
d) 4, 3,2,5,1
e) 4, 2,3,5,1

answer: d) 4, 3,2,5,1

15. The P wave of the electrocardiogram is a signal from
a) depolarization of the SA node
b) depolarization of the AV node
c) depolarization of the atria
d) repolarization of the atria
e) depolarization of the ventricles

answer: c) depolarization of the atria

16. Depolarization of the ventricles is represented on an electrocardiogram by the
a) P wave
b) T wave
c) S wave
d) QRS complex
e) PR complex

answer: d) QRS complex

17. Depolarization of the atria corresponds to the EKG's
a) P wave
b) QRS complex
c) QT interval
d) T wave
e) S-T segment

answer: a) P wave

18. Put in correct order the sequence in which excitation would move through the conducting system of the heart:
1. Purkinje fibers
2. AV bundle
3. AV node
4. SA node

5. bundle branches
a) 4, 3,2,5,1
b) 3, 5,4,2,1
c) 1, 4,3,2,5
d) 4, 2,3,5,1
e) 3, 2,4,5,1

answer: a) 4, 3,2,5,1

19. With each ventricular systole,
a) blood pressure remains steady
b) the ventricles fill with blood
c) blood pressure decreases
d) cardiac output decreases
e) blood pressure increases

answer: e) blood pressure increases

20. An increase in the rate of action potentials from baroreceptors will trigger a reflex to
a) increases in heart rate
b) decrease in heart rate
c) decrease in blood pressure
d) both decrease heart rate and decrease pressure
e) both increase heart rate and increase pressure

answer: d) both decreases heart rate and decrease pressure

21. The volume of blood ejected from each ventricle during a contraction is called the
a) end-diastolic volume
b) end-systolic volume
c) stroke volume
d) cardiac output
e) cardiac reserve

answer: c) stroke volume

22. Which of these would cause stroke volume to increase?
a) when venous return is decreased
b) when ventricular contraction is reduced
c) when diastolic blood pressure is decreased
d) decrease in heart rate
e) all of the answers are correct

answer: c) when diastolic blood pressure is decreased

23. Calculate the cardiac output of a patient with a heart rate of 100 beats/minute and a stroke volume of 75 ml.
a) 0.75 ml/ min
b) 750 ml/ min
c) 7500 ml/ min
d) 175 ml/ min
e) 25 ml/ min

answer: c) 7500 ml/ min

24. Compared to arteries, veins
a) are more elastic
b) have more smooth muscle in their tunica media
c) have a pleated endothelium
d) have thinner walls
e) hold their shape better when cut

answer: d) have thinner walls

25. Arrange the structures in the following list in the order that blood will encounter as it flows from the output side to the input side of the cardiovascular flow circuit
1. venules
2. arterioles
3. capillaries
4. elastic arteries
5. medium veins
6. large veins
7. muscular arteries
a) 7,4,2,3,1,5,6
b) 6,5,1,3,2,7,4
c) 5,6,1,3,2,7,4
d) 2,7,6,3,1,5,6
e) 4,7,2,3,1,5,6

answer: e) 4,7,2,3,1,5,6

26. Capillaries that have a complete lining are called
a) continuous capillaries
b) fenestrated capillaries
c) sinusoidal capillaries
d) sinusoids
e) vasa vasorum

answer: a) continuous capillaries

27. Venoconstriction _____ the amount of blood within the venous system, which _____ the volume in the arterial and capillary system
a) doubles; decreases
b) reduces; increases
c) decreases; doubles
d) increases; reduces
e) reduces; reduces

answer: b) reduces; increases

28. The layer of the arteriole wall that can produce vasoconstriction is the
a) tunica adventitia
b) tunica media
c) tunica intima
d) tunica externa
e) tunica master

answer: b) tunica media

29. These vessels may be continuous or fenestrated.
a) arteries
b) arterioles
c) capillaries
d) venules
e) veins

answer: c) capillaries

30. Capillaries with a perforated lining are called
a) perforated capillaries
b) discontinuous capillaries
c) fenestrated capillaries
d) sinuses
e) vasa vasorum

answer: c) fenestrated capillaries

31. Which of the following are the smallest venous vessels?
a) large veins
b) venules
c) medium veins
d) arteriovenules
e) venous valves

answer: b) venules

32. Which part of the vascular system functions as a blood reservoir and contains over 60% of the body's blood?
a) pulmonary
b) capillaries
c) systemic arterioles
d) veins
e) arteries

answer d) veins

33. List in correct order the sequence of blood vessels that blood would travel in the systemic circuit starting at the aorta.
1. venules
2. arterioles
3. capillaries
4. elastic arteries
5. medium veins
7. muscular arteries
a) 6,5,1,3,2,7,4
b) 4,7,2,3,1,5,6
c) 7,4,2,3,1,5,6
d) 5,6,1,3,2,7,4
e) 2,7,6,3,1,5,6

answer: b) 4,7,2,3,1,5,6

34. As blood travels from arteries to veins,
a) pressure builds
b) pressure drops
c) becomes turbulent
d) viscosity increases
e) diameter of the blood vessels gets progressively smaller

answer: e) diameter of the blood vessels gets progressively smaller

35. Which of the following factors will increase the net filtration pressure to move fluid out of capillaries?
a) decreased plasma albumen
b) increased blood hydrostatic pressure
c) increased tissue hydrostatic pressure
d) both decreased plasma albumin and increased blood hydrostatic pressure
e) increased plasma albumen

answer: d) both decreased plasma albumin and increased blood hydrostatic pressure

36. Which of the following affects blood flow through the body?
a) blood viscosity
b) vessel diameter
c) turbulence
d) vascular resistance
e) all of the answers are correct

answer: e) all of the answer are correct

37. The continual movement of fluid through the interstitial spaces produced by capillary filtration serves which of the following functions?
a) accelerates the distribution of nutrients and hormones
b) assist the transport of insoluble substances that cannot enter the capillaries
c) helps carry toxins and bacteria to the cell of the immune system
d) flushes hormones and wastes from the interstitial spaces
e) all of the answers are correct

answer: e) all of the answers are correct

38. The blood colloid osmotic pressure mostly depends on the
a) concentration of plasma sodium ions
b) concentration of plasma glucose
c) concentration of plasma waste products
d) concentration of plasma proteins
e) number of red blood cells

answer: d) concentration of plasma proteins

39. In comparison to a vessel with a large diameter, a vessels with a small diameter has
a) less resistance to blood flow
b) the same amount of pressure as resistance
c) a greater resistance to blood pressure
d) a higher blood pressure
e) a greater blood flow

answer: c) a greater resistance to blood pressure

40. As blood circulates from arteries into capillaries, the total cross-sectional are of capillaries
a) decreases and causes the blood velocity to decrease
b) is the same as the total cross-sectional area of arteries and blood velocity is equal between arteries and capillaries

c) increases and causes the blood velocity to decrease
d) increases and causes the blood velocity to increase
e) decreases and causes the blood velocity to increase

answer: c) increases and causes the blood velocity to decrease

41. Which of the following is normally the greatest source acting against blood flow?
a) vascular resistance
b) venous pressure
c) viscosity of blood
d) vessel length
e) turbulence

answer: a) vascular resistance

42. The force that move fluid out of capillaries is _____ pressure whereas the opposing force that moves fluid into capillaries is _____ pressure
a) systolic; diastolic
b) hydrostatic; osmotic
c) blood; interstitial
d) osmotic; hydrostatic
e) plasma; extracellular

answer: b) hydrostatic; osmotic

43. Some of the fluid that is forced out of capillaries is returned to the blood by the:
a) muscular arteries
b) liver
c) hepatic portal vein
d) venules
e) lymphatic system

answer: e) lymphatic system

44. Which of the following opposes the flow of blood back to the heart?
a) vascular resistance
b) peripheral veins have valves to prevent backflow of blood
c) muscular pumps squeeze veins and move blood toward the heart
d) blood pressure
e) blood pressure gradient from arteries to veins

answer: a) vascular resistance

45. To defend blood volume against dehydration, the body
a) accelerates reabsorption of water at the kidneys

b) experiences a recall of interstitial fluids
c) experiences an increase in the blood colloidal osmotic pressure
d) increases water intake
e) all of the answers are correct

answer: e) all of the answers are correct

Quiz 7

1) The primary function of the lymphatic system is
A) circulation of nutrients.
B) the transport of hormones.
C) defending the body against both environmental hazards and internal threats.
D) the production and distribution of plasma proteins.
E) circulation of dissolved gases.

answer: C) defending the body against both environmental hazards and internal threats

2) Compared to blood capillaries, lymph capillaries exhibit all of the following, except that they
A) have no basement membrane.
B) are larger in diameter.
C) have walls of endothelial cells that overlap like shingles.
D) are smaller in diameter.
E) are frequently irregular in shape.

answer: D) are smaller in diameter.

3) The cells directly responsible for cellular immunity are the _____ cells.
A) B
B) plasma
C) helper T
D) cytotoxic T
E) suppressor T

answer: D) cytotoxic T

4) The cells responsible for humoral immunity are the _____ cells.
A) NK
B) B
C) helper T
D) cytotoxic T
E) suppressor T

answer: B) B

5) Lymphocytes that destroy foreign cells or virus-infected cells are _____ cells.
A) B
B) plasma
C) helper T
D) cytotoxic T

E) suppressor T

answer: D) cytotoxic T

6) If the thymus shrank and stopped making thymosins, we would expect to see an immediate decrease in the number of
A) B lymphocytes.
B) NK cells.
C) T cells.
D) neutrophils.
E) red blood cells

answer: C) T cells

7) The body's innate defenses include all of the following, except
A) the skin.
B) complement.
C) interferon.
D) inflammation.
E) antibodies.

answer: E) antibodies

8) Each of the following is a physical barrier to infection, except
A) body hair.
B) epithelium.
C) secretions.
D) complement.
E) basement membranes

answer: D) complement

9) An inflammatory response is triggered when
A) red blood cells release pyrogens.
B) T cells release interferon.
C) mast cells release histamine and heparin.
D) neutrophils phagocytize bacteria.
E) blood flow to an area increases.

answer: C) mast cells release histamine and heparin

10) Inflammation produces localized
A) swelling.
B) redness.
C) heat.

D) pain.
E) All of the answers are correct

answer: E) all of the answers are correct

11) Leslie has a bad sore throat and the lymph nodes in her neck are swollen. This would indicate that
A) the focus of the infection is the lymph nodes.
B) lymph is not flowing through these lymph nodes.
C) the affected lymph nodes contain an increased number of lymphocytes.
D) the lymph node is actively producing phagocytes.
E) the lymph node has increased its secretion of thymosin.

answer: C) the affected lymph nodes contain an increased number of lymphocytes.

12) Cytotoxic T cells can attack target cells with which of these chemical weapons?
A) secrete strong acid
B) secrete organic solvent
C) secrete free radicals
D) secrete a cytokine that triggers apoptosis
E) secrete mutant proteins

answer: D) secrete a cytokine that triggers apoptosis

13) The following are steps in the cell-mediated immune response.
1. Several cycles of mitosis occur.
2. Antigen is engulfed and presented by a macrophage.
3. Cytotoxic T cells migrate to focus of infection.
4. T cells with specific receptors recognize the antigen.
5. T cells differentiate into cytotoxic T cells or T memory cells.
6. Cytotoxic T cells release perforin and/or lymphotoxin.
The correct sequence for these steps is
A) 4, 1, 5, 3, 6, 2
B) 2, 4, 1, 5, 3, 6.
C) 1, 2, 4, 5, 3, 6
D) 3, 2, 4, 1, 5, 6.
E) 3, 6, 4, 5, 1, 2

answer: B) 2, 4, 1, 5, 3, 6

14) When an antigen is bound to a Class I MHC molecule, it can stimulate a _____ cell.
A) B
B) plasma
C) helper T
D) cytotoxic T

E) NK

answer: D) cytotoxic T

15) When an antigen is bound to a Class II MHC protein, it can activate a _____ cell.
A) plasma
B) helper T
C) NK
D) suppressor T
E) cytotoxic T

answer: B) helper T

16) The C shape of the tracheal cartilages is important because
A) large masses of food can pass through the esophagus during swallowing.
B) large masses of air can pass through the trachea.
C) it facilitates turning of the head.
D) the bronchi are also C-shaped.
E) it permits the trachea to pinch shut prior to sneezing.

answer: A) large masses of food can pass through the esophagus during swallowing.

17) The following is a list of some airways of the respiratory system.
1. secondary bronchus
2. bronchioles
3. alveolar ducts
4. primary bronchus
5. respiratory bronchiole
6. alveoli
7. terminal bronchiole
The order in which air passes through is
A) 4, 1, 2, 7, 5, 3, 6
B) 4, 1, 2, 5, 7, 3, 6
C) 1, 4, 2, 5, 7, 3, 6
D) 1, 4, 2, 7, 5, 3, 6
E) 2, 4, 1, 7, 5, 3, 6.

answer: A) 4, 1, 2, 7, 5, 3, 6

18) The respiratory membrane of the gas exchange surfaces consists of
A) pseudostratified ciliated columnar epithelium.
B) moist cuboidal epithelium.
C) simple squamous epithelium.
D) ciliated squamous epithelium.
E) surfactant cells.

answer: C) simple squamous epithelium.

19) Which direction does carbon dioxide move during internal respiration?
A) from the blood into the tissue cells
B) from the blood into the lungs
C) from the lungs into the atmosphere
D) from the tissue cells into the blood
E) from the lungs into the blood

answer: D) from the tissue cells into the blood

20) If the volume of the lungs increases, what happens to the air pressure inside the lungs?
A) decreases
B) increases and possibly damages the lungs
C) increases twice the amount of the increase in volume
D) remains constant
E) increases

answer: A) decreases

21) When the diaphragm and external intercostal muscles contract,
A) the volume of the thorax increases.
B) the volume of the thorax decreases.
C) the volume of the lungs decreases.
D) the lungs shrink.
E) expiration occurs.

answer: A) the volume of the thorax increases.

22) Pulmonary ventilation refers to the
A) movement of air into and out of the lungs.
B) movement of dissolved gases from the alveoli to the blood.
C) movement of dissolved gases from the blood to the interstitial space.
D) movement of dissolved gases from the interstitial space to the cells.
E) utilization of oxygen.

answer: A) movement of air into and out of the lungs.

23) The function of pulmonary ventilation is to
A) remove carbon dioxide from the blood.
B) supply oxygen to the blood.
C) maintain adequate alveolar ventilation.
D) remove air from dead air space.
E) prevent gas exchange in the bronchioles

answer: C) maintain adequate alveolar ventilation.

24) Air moves out of the lungs when the pressure inside the lungs is
A) less than the pressure in the atmosphere.
B) greater than the pressure in the atmosphere.
C) equal to the pressure in the atmosphere.
D) greater than intraalveolar pressure.
E) less than intrapulmonic pressure.

answer: B) greater than the pressure in the atmosphere

25) Most of the oxygen transported by the blood is
A) dissolved in plasma.
B) bound to hemoglobin.
C) in ionic form as solute in the plasma.
D) bound to the same protein as carbon dioxide.
E) carried by white blood cells.

answer: B) bound to hemoglobin.

26) Most of the carbon dioxide in the blood is transported as
A) solute dissolved in the plasma.
B) carbaminohemoglobin.
C) bicarbonate ions.
D) solute dissolved in the cytoplasm of red blood cells.
E) carbonic acid.

answer: C) bicarbonate ions.

27) Which of the following factors would increase the amount of oxygen discharged by hemoglobin to peripheral tissues?
A) decreased temperature
B) decreased pH
C) increased tissue PO2
D) decreased amounts of DPG
E) All of the answers are correct.

answer: B) decreased pH

28) The most important chemical regulator of respiration is
A) oxygen.
B) carbon dioxide.
C) bicarbonate ion.
D) sodium ion.

E) hemoglobin

answer: B) carbon dioxide.

29) In quiet breathing,
A) inspiration and expiration involve muscular contractions.
B) inspiration is passive and expiration involves muscular contractions.
C) inspiration involves muscular contractions and expiration is passive.
D) inspiration and expiration are both passive.
E) inspiration is deep and forceful.

answer: C) inspiration involves muscular contractions and expiration is passive.

30) Blocking afferent action potentials from the chemoreceptors in the carotid and aortic bodies would interfere with the brain's ability to regulate breathing in response to
A) changes in PCO2.
B) changes in PO2.
C) changes in pH.
D) changes in blood pressure.
E) changes in PCO2, PO2, and pH.

answer: E) changes in PCO2, PO2, and pH.

31) Digestion refers to the
A) progressive dehydration of indigestible residue.
B) mechanical breakdown of food.
C) chemical breakdown of food.
D) mechanical and chemical breakdown of food.
E) All of the answers are correct.

answer: D) mechanical and chemical breakdown of food.

32) Waves of muscular contractions that propel the contents of the digestive tract are called
A) segmentation.
B) pendular movements.
C) peristalsis.
D) churning movements.
E) mastication.

answer: C) peristalsis.

33) A structure that helps prevent food from entering the pharynx prematurely is the
A) uvula.

B) pharyngeal arch.
C) palatoglossal arch.
D) palatopharyngeal arch.
E) epiglottis.

answer: A) uvula.

34) Which of the following is a function of the tongue?
A) manipulation to assist with chewing
B) mechanical processing
C) sensory analysis
D) secretion of mucins
E) All of the answers are correct.

answer: E) All of the answers are correct

35) The enzyme pepsin digests
A) carbohydrates.
B) proteins.
C) lipids.
D) nucleic acids.
E) vitamins.

answer: B) proteins.

36) The stomach is different from other digestive organs in that it
A) has folds in the mucosa.
B) has three layers of muscle in the muscularis externa.
C) secretes digestive juice.
D) moves by peristalsis.
E) secretes digestive hormones.

answer: B) has three layers of muscle in the muscularis externa

37) Plicae and intestinal villi
A) increase the surface area of the mucosa of the small intestine.
B) carry products of digestion that will not pass through the walls of blood capillaries.
C) produce new cells for the mucosa of the small intestine.
D) secrete digestive enzymes.
E) produce hormones.

answer: A) increase the surface area of the mucosa of the small intestine.

38) Which of these enhance the absorptive effectiveness of the small intestine?
A) the plicae circulares

B) the villi
C) the microvilli
D) intestinal movements
E) All of the answers are correct.

answer: E) All of the answers are correct.

39) Plicae circulares are
A) ridges in the wall of the stomach.
B) circumferential folds in the mucosa and submucosa of the small intestine.
C) fingerlike projections on the surface of the mucosa of the small intestine.
D) sacculations in the colon.
E) abnormal structures formed by excessive pressure in the small intestine.

answer: B) circumferential folds in the mucosa and submucosa of the small intestine.

40) The pancreas produces
A) lipases and amylase.
B) nucleases.
C) peptidases and proteinases.
D) sodium bicarbonate.
E) All of the answers are correct.

answer: E) All of the answers are correct

41) Bile is stored in the
A) liver.
B) duodenum.
C) pancreas.
D) gallbladder.
E) appendix.

answer: D) gallbladder.

42) Which digestive juice contains enzymes that breakdown carbohydrates, lipids, and proteins?
A) intestinal juice
B) pancreatic juice
C) bile
D) gastric juice
E) saliva

answer: B) pancreatic juice

43) Haustra are
A) expansible pouches of the colon.
B) strips of muscle in the colon.
C) glands in the large intestine that secrete mucus.
D) the source of colon hormones.
E) compact feces stored in the rectum.

answer: A) expansible pouches of the colon.

44) A small, wormlike structure attached to the posteromedial surface of the cecum is the
A) haustra.
B) pancreas.
C) gallbladder.
D) appendix.
E) ileum.

answer: D) appendix.

45) Carbohydrate digestion begins in the
A) mouth.
B) esophagus.
C) stomach.
D) duodenum.
E) ileum.

Answer A) Mouth

Medical Root Words

A

abdomin/o abdomen
acou/o hearing
aden/o gland
adenoid/o adenoids
adren/o adrenal gland
alveol/o alveolus
amni/o amnion
andro/o male
angi/o vessel
ankly/o stiff
anter/o frontal
an/o anus
aponeur/o aponeurosis
appendic/o appendix
arche/o beginning
arteri/o artery
atri/o atrium
aur/i ear
aur/o ear
aut/o self

B

bacteri/o bacteria
balan/o glans penis
bi/o life
blephar/o eyelid
bronch/i bronchus
bronch/o bronchus

C

calc/i calcium
cancer/o cancer
carcin/o cancer
cardi/o heart
carp/o carpals
caud/o tail
cec/o cecum
celi/o abdomen
cephal/o head
cerebell/o cerebellum
cerebr/o cerebrum
cervic/o cervix
cheil/o lip
cholangi/o bile duct
.chol/e gall
chondro/o cartilage
chori/o chorion
chrom/o color
clavic/o clavicle
col/o colon
colp/o vagina
core/o pupil
corne/o cornea
coron/o heart
cortic/o cortex
cor/o pupil
cost/o rib
crani/o cranium
cry/o cold
cutane/o skin
cyes/i pregnancy
cyst/o bladder

D

dacry/o tear
dermat/o skin
diaphragmat/o diaphragm
dipl/o double
dips/o thirst
dist/o distal
diverticul/o diverticulum
dors/o back
duoden/o duodenum
dur/o dura

E

ech/o sound
electr/o electricity
embry/o embryo
encephal/o brain
endocrin/o endocrine
enter/o intestine
epididym/o epididymis
epiglott/o epiglottis
episi/o vulva
epitheli/o epithelium
erythr/o red
esophag/o esophagus
esthesi/o sensation

F

femor/o femur
fet/i fetus
fet/o fetus
fibr/o fibrous tissue
fibul/o fibula

G

ganglion/o ganglion
gastr/o stomach
gingiv/o gum
glomerul/o glomerulus
gloss/o tongue
glyc/o sugar
gnos/o knowledge
gravid/o pregnancy
gynec/o woman

H

hem/o blood
hepat/o liver
herni/o hernia
heter/o other
hidr/o sweat
hist/o tissue
humer/o humerus
hydr/o water
hymen/o hymen
hyster/o uterus

I

ile/o ileum
ili/o ilium
irid/o iris
iri/o iris
ischi/o ischium
ischo/o blockage

J

jejun/o jejunum

K

kal/i potassium
kary/o nucleus
kerat/o hard
kinesi/o motion
kyph/o hump

L

lacrim/o tear duct
lact/o milk
lamin/o lamina
lapar/o abdomen
later/o lateral
lei/o smooth
leuk/o white
lingu/o tongue
lip/o fat

lith/o stone
lob/o lob/o
lord/o flexed forward
lumb/o lumbar
lymph/o lymph

M

mamm/o breast
mandibul/o mandible
mast/o breast
mastoid/o mastoid
maxill/o maxilla
meat/o opening
melan/o black
mening/o meninges
menisc/o meniscus
men/o menstruation
ment/o mind
metr/i uterus
metr/o uterus
mon/o one
muc/o mucus
myc/o fungus
myel/o spinal cord
my/o muscle

N

nas/o nose
nat/o birth
necr/o death
nephr/o kidney
neur/o nerve
noct/i night

O

ocul/o eye
olig/o few
omphal/o navel
onc/o tumor
onych/o nail
oophor/o ovary
ophthalm/o eye
opt/o vision

orchid/o testicle
orch/o testicle
organ/o organ
or/o mouth
orth/o straight
oste/o bone
ot/o ear
ox/i oxygen

P

pachy/o thick
palat/o palate
pancreat/o pancreas
par/o labor
patell/o patella
path/o disease
pelv/i pelvis
perine/o peritoneum
petr/o stone
phalang/o pharynx
phas/o speech
phleb/o vein
phot/o light
phren/o mind
plasm/o plasma
pleur/o pleura
pneumon/o lung
poli/o gray matter
polyp/o small growth
poster/o posterior
prim/i first
proct/o rectum
proxim/o proximal
pseud/o fake
psych/o mind
pub/o pubis
puerper/o childbirth
pulmon/o lung
pupill/o pupil
pyel/o renal pelvis
pylor/o pylorus
py/o pus

Q

quadr/i four

R
rachi/o spinal
radic/o nerve
radi/o radius
rect/o rectum
ren/o kidney
retin/o retina
rhabd/o striated
rhytid/o wrinkles
rhiz/o nerve

S

sacr/o sacrum
scapul/o scapula
scler/o sclera
scoli/o curved
seb/o sebum
sept/o septum
sial/o saliva
sinus/o sinus
somat/o body
son/o sound
spermat/o sperm
spir/o breathe
splen/o spleen
spondyl/o vertebra
staped/o stapes
staphyl/o clusters
stern/o sternum
steth/o chest
stomat/o mouth
strept/o chain-like
super/o superior
synovi/o synovia

T
tars/o tarsal
ten/o tendon
test/o testicle
therm/o heat
thorac/o thorax
thromb/o clot

thym/o thymus
thyroid/o thyroid gland
tibi/o tibia
tom/o pressure
tonsill/o tonsils
toxic/o poison
trachel/o trachea
trich/o hair
tympan/o eardrum

U

uln/o ulna
ungu/o nail
ureter/o ureter
urethr/o urethra
ur/o urine
uter/o uterus
uvul/o uvula

V

vagin/o vagina
valv/o valve
vas/o vessel
ven/o vein
ventricul/o ventricle
ventro/o frontal
vertebr/o vertebra
vesic/o bladder
vesicul/o seminal vesicle

Prefixes

an- without
ante- before
bi- two
brady- slow
dia- through
dys- difficult
endo- within
epi- over
eu- normal
exo- outward
hemi- half
hyper- excessive
hypo- deficient
inter- between
intra- within
meta- change
multi- numerous
nulli- none
pan- total
para- beyond
per- through
peri- surrounding
post- after
pre- before
pro- before
sub- below
supra- superior
sym- join
syn- join
tachy- rapid
tetra- four
trans- through

Suffixes

-al pertaining to
-algia pain
-apheresis removal
-ary pertaining to
-asthenia weakness
-capnia carbon dioxide
-cele hernia
-clasia break
-clasis break
-crit separate
-cyte cell
-desis fusion
-drome run
-eal pertaining to
-ectasis expansion
-ectomy removal
-esis condition
-genesis cause
-genic pertaining to
-gram record
-graph recording device
-ial pertaining to
-iasis condition
-iatrist physician
-iatry specialty
-ic pertaining to
-ician one that
-ictal attack
-ior pertaining to
-ism condition of
-itis inflammation
-lysis separating
-malacia softening
-meter measure
-odynia pain
-oid resembling
-ology study
-oma tumor
-opia vision
-opsy view of
-orrhaphy repairing
-orrhea flow
-osis condition
-otomy cut into
-oxia oxygen
-paresis partial paralysis
-pathy disease
-pepsia digestion
-pexy suspension
-phagia swallowing, eating
-phobia excessive fear of
-phonia sound, voice
-physis growth
-plasia development
-plasm a growth
-plegia paralysis
-pnea breathing
-poiesis formation
-ptosis sagging
-salpinx fallopian tube
-sacoma malignant tumor
-schisis crack
-sclerosis hardening
-stasis standing
-stenosis narrowing
-thorax chest
-tocia labor, birth
-tome cutting device
-trophy develop
-uria urine

Printed in Great Britain
by Amazon